SOMEBODY TOLD ME I COULD

A POLIO SURVIVOR WHO'S IN IT FOR THE LONG HAUL

DIANNE MCTAGGART WALL

STRONG ANAM LLC

SOMEBODY TOLD ME I COULD
A Polio Survivor Who's In It For The Long Haul
by
Dianne McTaggart Wall
Published by Strong Anam, LLC
P.O. Box 195220
Winter Springs, FL 32719-5220
First edition, 2022
© Copyright 2022 Dianne M. Wall, All rights reserved.
Ebook ISBN 979-8-9867102-0-4
Paperback ISBN 979-8-9867102-1-1
Library of Congress Control Number: 2022923115
Printed in the United States of America

The stories in this book reflect the author's recollection of events. Some names, locations, and identifying characteristics have been changed to protect the privacy of those depicted. Dialogue has been re-created from memory.

I dedicate this book to Dennis and Katie, the BIGGEST "Somebodies" in my life.

INTRODUCTION

I was born with a virus during an epidemic. It would have been a pandemic if people had not gotten vaccinated.

The polio epidemic was eventually controlled by a high distribution of vaccines. High vaccination rates prevent epidemics from becoming pandemics. However, when I was born with the polio virus in 1953, the world was still waiting for an available vaccine.

The polio vaccine was still in its discovery and testing phase in 1953. If the vaccine was available then, my mother would have gotten it to protect me and everyone else around her. Parents today have that choice—a choice my mother did not have. People can choose to protect their children, born and unborn, by getting vaccinated. Without that choice, my mother was one of the thousands who contracted polio that year. Without a viable vaccine, I was born with polio and now live with Post-Polio Syndrome, more commonly referred to as PPS.

While writing this story, I'm thinking about many people I have met recently— ones who say, "What's polio?" Unfortunately, some of them are in the medical field! To answer their question, you should know some history.

Normal, everyday living stopped where the polio virus struck. Thousands of people, of all ages, were crippled or killed. Many of them were children. Places where people would gather for recreation were closed. Parks with picnic areas, lakes and community swimming pools, theaters, and even churches were shut down. People were very scared of catching polio. Many thought it could be acquired and spread quickly with any human contact. Neighbors turned on each other if a family was known to have contracted polio. Fear of the disease had hit all walks of life—even a President of the United States. The virus drove families to protect themselves at all costs. Some chose to keep their houses shut up tightly, all windows and doors closed no matter how hot it was.

Many major polio epidemics took place in very warm weather, at a time when families loved to cool off in the water. Many epidemics were found to spread quickly at neighborhood pools and lakes.

It wasn't until 1952 that a vaccine was developed. It took another 3 years before the vaccine started to be distributed, in 1955. When I was born in 1953, the threat of polio was very real. After my mom contracted polio, it required a giant leap of faith by my family and neighbors to even think of coming near her.

Several years ago when I was visiting my hometown of Elkader, Iowa, I spoke with one of those neighbors. She told me. "Oh honey, I'll never forget my husband coming home from a visit with your dad. He came into the house and just sat down and cried. Being just across the street, we heard the commotion the night before and saw the doctor make a house call. We knew something was wrong, but we didn't want to be too nosy." She then said, "It was from that visit when we all learned about your mom getting polio. Both of us started crying when we looked at each other and thought; *how in the world could your mom deliver you?*"

It was from that short visit that the neighborhood found out polio had come to Elkader. It had hit my mom, and me too.

My neighbor continued, "We wondered what would happen to your dad and the kids. We were scared about our family's exposure to polio too." The very real threat of polio had just entered their world.

Thanks to the vaccine, I'm happy to report the polio virus has been eradicated in most parts of the world today. This leads me to think about the many young parents today who are against vaccinating their child. They see polio vaccination as just one more shot on the doctor's list. They have no knowledge of what their choice can mean for their child. The consequence of their choice can lead to permanent damage to their child's brain stem, which can lead to paralysis and a lifelong disability. These young parents may never be told what polio was, and still is. As I said earlier, some of today's medical professionals don't even know their polio history, so how can young parents be medically advised?

As I write these words, it is the spring of 2021. For over a year we have been living through a worldwide pandemic of COVID-19. Parents can protect their children from the current coronavirus. They can protect their children with a vaccine that has proven effective against sickness and death. There are never any good arguments as to why parents should not protect their own children if they can. Parents shouldn't let their own prejudices get in the way when it comes to the safety of their children.

I have had doctors tell me that no one can be born with polio, or in medical terminology, "polio in utero." But I was. I have read some papers written by medical experts, that are adamantly certain that my story of "polio in utero" is IMPOSSIBLE! I have learned that doctors don't know everything.

I can't tell you how many doctors have asked me, "How do you do that?" They ask that question about a huge array of everyday tasks people do without blinking an eye. How do I walk? How do I get dressed? How do I brush my hair or my teeth? How do I get up from a toilet? How do I drive? I'd love to explain how I make love, but none of them ever asked me that.

When doctors look at my history and learn I'm a musician with a master's degree in music therapy, they find out that I sing, play guitar and piano. In addition to daily life questions, they then ask: "How do you play guitar? How do you play piano, since you have never been able to raise your arms above your waist? How can you sing with your severe scoliosis squeezing your diaphragm and lungs?" . . . . .etc. etc. etc. I have to admit that I love to demonstrate how I sing—being shy is just not part of my DNA. Then I love watching their faces!

These days, PPS has changed some of my answers to how I do what I do. Adapting my methods to accommodate the many weaknesses throughout my body has taken a toll on my joints. As polio survivors age, we lose some of our favorite "can-do methods" that we perfected to get the job done. However, I will explain more on PPS later in my story.

I can definitely say that I have been blessed with some terrific doctors in my lifetime. Okay, in full disclosure here, I've had some NOT so terrific ones too, but I've fixed that by just firing them! However, the good ones I keep, like my very first one, Dr. Ignacio Ponseti, who was a world-renowned orthopedic surgeon. Do an internet search on him and you will know how blessed I was having him as my doctor. There is a New York Times obituary written by Douglas Martin, dated October 24, 2009 titled, "Dr. Ignacio Ponseti, Hero to Many with Clubfoot, Dies at 95." It gives the historical account of Dr. Ponseti's life, but it also explains the orthopedic method he developed that changed the orthopedic world of surgical intervention.

Another physician who's a "keeper" is my physiatrist Dr. Mitchell Freed, who specializes in physical rehabilitation. He has followed me with excellent medical care for over 20 years. Not only is he an extremely talented doctor, but he is one of the most patient and compassionate people I have ever known. Both Dr. Ponseti and Dr. Freed practiced the philosophy that good doctors are always "practicing" medicine while treating me. When they didn't have an exact fix to help me, they used their "practice" methods based on their solid medical knowledge. Then they came up with answers that allowed me to thrive. As a musical child, and now as an adult musician, I can say that I have always related to the phrase, "practice makes perfect."

For years I would hear my doctors' questions about how I walk, brush my hair, and do all the ordinary, daily living-skills we all do. I always answered with, "I don't know how I do them, I just do them." I was reflecting on those questions recently, while I was recuperating from one of my many falls, which I prefer to call stunts. This particular stunt was the fourth time that I split my left kneecap. While sitting in my wheelchair with my splinted leg extended, it finally came to me: I should answer those doctors' questions with the statement, "Somebody told me I could!"

This is my story of those special "somebodies" and how their faith in me shaped my absolutely wonderful life. I have no doubt I will meet more "somebodies" who will tell me that I can!

1

I'll begin my story with the first "somebodies that told me I could." First my mom, Virginia, and my dad, Bill. They were raised Catholic, and they relied on their faith to see them through life's trials and tribulations. My siblings and I were raised Catholic as well. However, to say that my deep faith was mined only from the catechism I was taught would not be true. My faith is the result of both my religious upbringing and the life I have led. To understand my story, you will need to keep that in mind. My faith is my own, and it has been created, shaped and reaffirmed time and again by my own experiences.

In the following narrative, my parents, grandmothers, uncles, aunts, siblings and neighbors are described in a sequence of life events. I have recreated these events as faithfully as possible, based on oral history, family stories and conversations with relatives and friends. It is with love that I offer up this account of those events that transpired when I was very young or before I was born. These events built the foundation of my life, and they made all the difference.

. . .

VIRGINIA COULDN'T SLEEP and she felt the baby moving. How could anyone sleep in this 95- degree heat. Iowa in late August and early September had some real heat spell doozies, but this one in 1953 had already lasted more than the usual three or four days. This heatwave was going on seven days now. That rarely happened.

Earlier that day, Virginia and Bill decided to go for a Labor Day weekend picnic. They packed up the station wagon with their two young kids, Pat who was four-year-old, and seventeen-month-old Colleen. Off they drove thirty miles from home to a nearby state park.

Taking a family picnic meant a lot of work for Virginia, getting all the food and drinks, towels, toys, and of course diapers for Colleen. But just the thought of splashing in cool water made all those chores worth it. Hard work was something Virginia always accepted, even as a very young child. She was raised during the Great Depression by her widowed mother, a tiny Irish woman who weighed no more than 100 pounds wet. Virginia grew up having that same petite stature. All through her school-aged years Virginia's schoolmates nicknamed her "bones." Even as frail as she looked, she was determined to help her mother. Virginia got her first paying job at the age of 8, delivering newspapers, and held that job until she was in high school, when she became the stock girl at the local dime store.

Still lying in bed, struggling to get comfortable, Virginia tried to center her thoughts of earlier that day. She remembered walking into the lake and embracing the wet relief. Her pregnant body's thermostat lowered as she entered the crowded lake. The water was almost as warm as bath water, but it still felt good. Even as petite as she was, she felt like a beached whale in her bathing suit. However, Virginia didn't care that the water wasn't actually cold and that there were a hundred or more families that had the same "cool" idea of swimming in the lake. After a short while of dodging many kids horsing around, it became a little too crowded for both Bill and Virginia. They decided to move to another good spot in the picnic area with a creek where the kids could safely splash around with less elbow jabbing. Being less crowded, they could all relax in the water. It was so nice to sit in the creek and feel the gentle flowing water cover her third-trimester-sized belly. No, she didn't care what she looked like. She was only aware of how the floating and weightlessness felt as she approached her due date three weeks away.

The next day was Labor Day September 7, 1953. Labor Day was then, and still is now the official closing of the swimming area at most parks. Virginia knew it was now or never to give herself that perfect weightless treat.

Although her friends had warned her of the dangers of swimming in public places during the height of polio season, this last trimester was so uncomfortable. This was her first pregnancy, and everything was new. Yes, she was already a mother, but Pat and Colleen were adopted, so being pregnant was one of the many firsts in her life.

Both Virginia and Bill had shared their desire to be parents before they were married, but having children was much more important to Virginia than it was to Bill. She once confided in her parish priest that she was worried she couldn't get pregnant, since she and Bill had been trying for the first four years of marriage yet still had no children. Father Ralph suggested they would be a perfect couple to consider adopting children. He offered to begin the process for them through an adoption agency. However, Virginia never told Bill that she had talked to the priest about her concerns and desires to be a mom. Well, that changed once she heard from Father Ralph several weeks after their meeting.

Father Ralph came to the house one night to give them the good news. A baby boy would be theirs to adopt if they would interview with the adoption agency. When Bill heard this, he felt he was ambushed by his wife and his own parish priest. As Father Ralph looked at the couple, he suspected Virginia had never told Bill about their talk. "I'll leave now so the two of you can discuss this opportunity," Father Ralph said as he quickly went out the door.

Bill was livid. He let Virginia know exactly what he was thinking and feeling. Adoption was a huge step and one they had never even discussed. He looked at Virginia and asked, "Why would you talk to the priest first and not to me? After all, I would be the child's father, not Father Ralph." In a very rare moment Virginia was speechless. Bill could see Virginia was devastated by his reaction, so he agreed, "Honey, I can see how much this means to you, so I'll agree to adopting."

So that was the beginning of the McTaggart family. Bill and Virginia adopted a boy first, who they named Pat, and then they adopted a baby girl who they named Colleen. They planned their family perfectly with their adopted children just 3 years apart, one of each sex. Well it was perfect timing until nine months after adopting Colleen, God made new plans—the family of three would later grow into a family of five!

While the unexpectedly pregnant Virginia lay in bed trying to get comfortable in the unprecedented heat of September 1953, the big window fan was blowing on high. The air should have been cooling her off, but it felt more like a blast from a furnace vent. No wonder the baby was kicking. Her body temperature was rising, and she was wringing wet with sweat. Bill was already snoring, and she marveled at how he could be so comfortable while they were both being baked alive. Then Virginia remembered that Bill loved to keep his case of cold beer in the cellar fridge. Bill reduced his beer supply quite a bit during the hot spell, but the fridge was cold and nothing else mattered that night. "Ahhhh," Virginia thought, "to be able to have a cold beer after September 28th, my due date."

It would not come soon enough for her. Would she have a boy or a girl? They had talked about naming a boy Michael, after Bill's dad. If it was a girl, they would use her family name for girls, Mary, like her parents used for her. Everyone called her Virginia though, because there were too many Marys in the family line. Since it was confusing at family gatherings, Virginia she became. Oh, to have a little Mary would be so precious, but a Michael would be wonderful too. Whichever, a boy or a girl, the baby sure could kick and especially at night! Virginia knew the baby didn't like this heat spell any more than she did.

She lay there rubbing her belly remembering how wonderful the cool water felt and how effortless it was to move. The baby didn't kick the whole time in the water. She imagined her baby might be a great swimmer, or a super-fast roller-skater, just like she was as a young girl. She recalled the breeze on her face as she roller-skated down the hills in their tiny Iowa town. Elkader was known as the Little Switzerland of Iowa. Hills were everywhere, and oh how she loved rolling down as fast as she could. Of course, having all these thoughts was not helping her get to sleep—her top priority. After all, she was a mother of a very active seventeen-month-old girl and a toddler who was all boy. She decided to turn her mind off by praying to the Blessed Mother. Mary Virginia knew her namesake would come to her aid, granting her the sleep she so desperately needed. Her prayers were answered, and she finally drifted off.

∼

IT WAS the late 1940's when my dad and mom bought their old three-story house with its thirteen rooms. They were young with lots of future renovations to look forward to. However, they never dreamt how hot they'd be in the summer and how frozen they'd be in the winter. In the 1940's and 50's, modern conveniences like central heat and air were only for the wealthy, and they were definitely not wealthy. While they dreamed about fixing it up as the years went by, their nearly 100-year-old house was a huge "money-pit." Mom knew that she and Dad were scraping by as it was. With two young children and a third on its way, Dad working at the family store wasn't going to make those dreams come true anytime soon.

The store was McTaggart and Sons Furniture Store, which

was started by my dad's mother Louise. She was better known as Lizzie Brinkhous McTaggart, after marrying Michael McTaggart. Dad began working full-time at the store right after he came back from the war. So did my uncle, Dad's older brother Don.

All of Grandma Lizzie and Grandpa Michael's five children had shared a terrible strain of influenza during childhood, and every one of them had had high fevers and respiratory complications. Their baby girl, Joanne, died of the influenza at the age of three. All three of the surviving McTaggart children, Dad, his other sister Luella, and his older brother Francis were all later afflicted with hearing problems. Uncle Don was the only one who completely recovered. Dad and Aunt Luella were just hard of hearing in one ear, but Francis, better known as Uncle Alvie, was severely hearing impaired.

Grandma Lizzie was quite the businesswoman, and one stubborn boss. Everyone knew she ran the business like a five-star general, and only her orders stood. She was brought up in the tiny township of Mederville, where her parents ran the Brinkhous General Store. It was the only store in town.

Almost everyone who settled in Mederville was German, and they took a lot of pride in how their houses and family businesses looked, and how they were run. The township was considered the German settlement of Clayton County.

Across the creek that ran nearby was the Irish settlement, Cox Creek township. The hard-working Irish that settled in Cox Creek were just as proud as their German neighbors. They made their homes with a scrappy determination mixed with a fighting Irish spirit. Both settlements were filled with hard-working, stubborn people that were determined to make their townships the very best they could be. The proud people of Mederville considered Cox Creek the other side of the tracks, and never should the two meet. But Lizzie Brinkhous of Mederville met Michael McTaggart of Cox Creek, fell in love, and thus began the McTaggart family and the family business, McTaggart and Sons' Furniture store.

VIRGINIA WAS THRASHING around trying to get comfortable and woke up shivering. How could she be so cold on such a blistering night? She realized that she was feverish, and her legs were throbbing with pain. She had never felt anything like this before. Her breathing was very labored, and parts of her body ached with painful muscle spasms. Was this what labor was supposed to feel like? She couldn't feel the baby move. She began to worry about the baby being so still. She looked to see what time it was. One o'clock in the morning. She had only been asleep for about three hours. She was frightened and woke Bill up. When he touched her forehead, and her arms and legs, she was burning up. All she wanted was more blankets so she could stop shaking from the chills. Bill knew this was the sickest he had ever seen Virginia, so he telephoned the town doctor, and explained her symptoms. Doc Smith told Bill that he would be right over. House calls were the norm back then, especially in small towns. Bill had never had to make an emergency call to Doc Smith for his wife before, just for the kids. Bill wondered if she was having complications with the pregnancy, since the due date was just three weeks away. He'd never experienced labor either, so he was relieved that Doc was on his way.

Bill knew Virginia was way too sick to take care of Pat and Colleen, both being toddlers, even if there was something that could break her fever. He also thought he might need help that very same night since the kids would probably wake up when Doc Smith arrived. Of course he'd wait to hear what Doc thought about how bad Virginia was. However, if help would be needed, he knew he'd call Aunt Winnie. She was Virginia's aunt who lived with Virginia's Mom, Ella. Aunt Winnie was really like another mom to the family and thankfully was just minutes away. Ella was a wonderful grandma in every way, but she had fallen and broken her hip a few years back, so

Winnie was the logical choice to help out. Bill listened to Virginia moaning and thrashing around while waiting for Doc Smith to arrive. Although everyone in town lived just minutes from each other, it felt like Doc lived five hours not five minutes away. It was the longest wait Bill had ever had for a house call, but he was relieved knowing help was coming.

Doc let himself in and went right up to their bedroom. Nobody ever locked their doors in town. Doc knew the layout of the house from responding to previous middle-of-the-night telephone calls from a nervous new mother. Bill acknowledged Doc when he walked in with his black medical bag in hand. Yet even with feeling the relief of Doc's arrival, Bill couldn't speak. He just kept his eyes on Virginia's shivering and feverish body.

Doc got right down to business examining her. Virginia started to scream when her legs were checked. Bill didn't feel his worries lessen as he hoped he would. Doc quietly noted Virginia's severe fever and chills, but when Doc looked at Virginia's legs, the muscles were twisting into terrible spasms. Her breathing was very shallow and her heart was racing. The thermometer read 104 degrees. He listened to the baby, and heard a heartbeat, but something seemed very odd in the baby's position. This was definitely not pregnancy complications or early labor. His suspicions would have to be investigated with medical tests that could be done only in a hospital. Elkader didn't have a hospital, and the nearest one was about 40 miles away. It was ironic, but Bill was one of the town ambulance drivers. However, he was in no shape to drive Virginia.

Bill's brother Don was called to be the backup driver. Furniture stores had funeral homes attached to them back in the day, and McTaggart & Sons Furniture was no different. The funeral home used a big station wagon for their hearse, with its back seats folded down. It was perfect to carry a gurney, transporting bodies. However, since the town had no hospital, their station wagon became a town ambulance as well, getting people to the closest hospitals available. The funeral home gurney was used for both the living and the dead, thus making Bill and Don town ambulance drivers, as well as undertakers.

While Doc Smith was working on Virginia, Bill made all the necessary telephone calls and got dressed. There was so much to think about. First was babysitting coverage for Pat and Colleen, so he made his planned call to Aunt Winnie. He knew she would come and stay at the house for as long as it might take. Since Aunt Winnie did not drive, Bill had to wait for her to call back to let him know when she would be ready. Second, Bill had to arrange transport for Virginia to the hospital. He knew he wasn't in the right frame of mind to drive the ambulance, so he called his brother Don. Once the ambulance and gurney were ready, Don would pick up Aunt Winnie.

Don knew he'd need help with the gurney, knowing his brother Bill was scared to death about Virginia. He recruited his next-door neighbor Ted and told him to go over to Bill and Virginia's house to wait for him there. Fortunately, Don lived with his mother Lizzie right across the street from Bill and Virginia's house. It was easy to get help quickly with everyone living so close to each other.

Don and Ted assisted Bill lifting the gurney, with Virginia in it. She was delirious and couldn't walk by the time they got her placed on the gurney to transport. They carefully carried her down the flight of stairs. Young Pat and Colleen had woken up with all the commotion. Aunt Winnie got them settled down. She knew she would be taking care of the kids for quite a while, for she knew her niece was in serious trouble. Aunt Winnie was ready to start her Rosaries that very night once the children were back in bed. Everyone was scared, but the one who was scared the most was Doc Smith.

∼

DOC SMITH WAS HOPING against hope that Virginia McTaggart had not picked up the polio virus while swimming at the state park earlier that day. He suspected that it was a strong possibility though—that polio had struck.

It was a well-known fact that polio could be transmitted very easily in highly congested public areas like parks. On this day in particular, the danger was great because of the combination of high heat and bodies of water. Summertime meant polio in the early 1950's. Entire towns feared that an outbreak would strike.

Most family doctors recognized polio symptoms when they saw them, and Doc Smith was no exception. He had delivered many babies in his practice, but he had never had an expectant mother come down with polio before.

By the time Virginia arrived at the hospital, her fever had gone up to 105 degrees. Doc Smith ordered a spinal tap which was the definitive test needed to properly diagnose polio. Oh, how he wished that Virginia had not gone swimming.

If the results of the spinal tap came back positive, he knew he would have to save the baby, though it would be almost a month premature. The thought of what could happen to Virginia and her newborn concerned him far more than he wanted to admit. He knew time was critical. He was also keenly aware that the baby's position had changed from where it should have been. In fact, when he examined Virginia's belly that night, he saw bulging areas that could only be from the infant's limbs pushing out. He had never seen anything like that before.

In the meantime, Bill was frantically pacing in the emergency room waiting room with Don and his neighbor Ted. All three of them knew from their forty-minute drive to the hospital that Virginia was fighting for her life. None of them understood why, since her symptoms didn't match anything like labor pains. Bill felt like this was a bad dream, and he wished he could wake up and it would be over. He was so thankful for not being alone during this nightmare, and more than once mentioned that to Don and Ted.

Don had been around many critically ill patients as a medic in

WWII, and he couldn't help but recognize danger in Virginia's moans as he drove the makeshift ambulance that evening. He knew not to mention any of his fears to his brother during this wait-and-see period. This was the time to pray and wait for the doctors and nurses to work their magic through the night on Virginia's feverish body. Don knew his tiny sister-in-law as a feisty, Irish woman. At times she got on his nerves, but right now he thought that her spunk would work in her favor—fighting for her life.

Several hours passed and Doc Smith came out to the waiting area. He was glad he found only the three people: Dad, Don and his neighbor Ted. Delivering the kind of news he had to deliver, he didn't need any bigger audience. He looked straight at Bill and told him the spinal tap was positive and Virginia had contracted polio. Doc explained that time was of the essence. Labor had to be induced so he could try to save both Virginia and the baby. He then explained that, once the baby was delivered, the hospital did not have the medical team necessary to treat the premature baby, who in his medical opinion, could be very compromised from Virginia's high fever and virus. Doc Smith knew that Ted's wife Lily, was a registered nurse, so he told Ted to call and tell her to drive to the hospital. She would be needed to hold the newborn baby during transport, as Don drove them to the closest teaching hospital which was over an hour away.

While Ted ran down the hall to the nearest telephone, Bill just stood there with a blank look on his face. He appeared to be in total shock. This wasn't what he and Virginia ever dreamed of when they got the news that Virginia was expecting. He had imagined waiting like other expectant fathers passing out cigars with his friends and family. Now it was going to take all the faith and courage he could muster to get through the next few hours. If there was one thing he knew for sure, it was that his wife was one heck of a fighter, as well as a true believer in the power of God. He also knew that if Doc Smith believed that this was the only way to save the lives of his wife and newborn baby, then his faith in God had to be his anchor and his trust had to be in Doc Smith.

~

HOURS PASSED and still no word from the nurses that walked by the waiting room. Bill read and reread every newspaper that was lying around. It wasn't easy for him to look like he was actually reading, because only he knew he had trouble comprehending the written word. He was a wizard with numbers, which is why he was good at going out on the carpeting and drapery orders for the store. Reading a paper for him meant looking at the stock market charts and judging the good and the bad advertising sections. He had noticed a furniture ad that used a picture of Diana the Goddess of Beauty in it, and he thought that was a clever hook for quality furniture. Bill was a natural businessman and very good with people, but when it came to reading words, his mind always got overloaded. Of course years later, the medical world would define Bill's problem as a learning disability called dyslexia. In the meantime, Bill successfully adapted his skills to meet life's demands.

At long last, a nurse came out still in her scrubs. She went directly to Bill and pulled her surgery mask down "The doctor just delivered your baby girl. Your wife is still feverish but stable. However, I need to know what name you and your wife want to name a baby girl?" Both she and the doctor were Catholics, like Bill, and knew that Catholics could perform Baptism in emergency situations. She then said, "Doc Smith wants to baptize your baby right away because he is not sure she will live long. The delivery was a very difficult one and he had to use forceps around the baby's head. Even though Virginia tried with all of her strength to bear down and push, she just couldn't."

Once again Bill felt shock, and he couldn't think of the names they had discussed, but the nurse insisted on a name and demanded the answer be fast. Bill said the first name he could remember, Dianne, which was his own spelling, from the furniture ad he had just seen in the newspaper. The nurse then asked for the middle name, needed for the Catholic baptismal tradition. It was only after she asked for the middle name that Bill remembered they were going to name the baby Mary, after Virginia's real first name of course. He decided that Dianne Mary would have to do. The nurse ran straight back to the delivery room as fast as lightning, before Bill had a chance to change the names.

Once Doc had successfully pulled the baby out, he saw and understood perfectly why Virginia could have never pushed her baby out naturally. The baby was totally paralyzed. Her little legs were frozen in a frog-like position. Her arms were bent up at the elbows. Her spine was severely twisted. Her head was paralyzed to one side. Baptism had to be performed quickly, for he did not think the baby would live.

Within the next half-hour, Doc Smith came out and explained to Bill that he felt Virginia was going to make it, but she was still in very critical condition. He was happy to report that it didn't appear that polio had caused any paralysis in her, but that baby Dianne was also in critical condition and needed a specialty team of doctors from the closest teaching hospital that was several miles away.

Doc Smith was glad he had made the decision to rush the baby to the specialized hospital. Uncle Don was ready and waiting with the car. The delivery nurse was preparing the infant and gathering provisions for the special needs during the hour-long transport. It would take a trained medical professional to know the emergency steps to engage during the transport, and the small hospital did not have extra staff to go along with the baby.

The child's life was delicately balancing between life and death, and nobody knew which way it would go during the next several hours. The delivery nurse was never so relieved to learn that the family friend Lily was a trained registered nurse. Everyone knew that keeping the baby warm would be important, but how in the world was Lily going to hold the poor, twisted tiny body that barely weighed

5 pounds and keep her alive? Doc Smith wished there had been an incubator that could have been used for the hour-long drive, but there wasn't any way of powering it up electrically.

Oxygen tubing and IV tubing were already attached to the baby, so the delivery team escorted Lily out with the IV bags and one transportable oxygen tank, which they set up in the back of the station wagon. Lily wrapped baby Dianne up warmly and held on to her carefully, while Don drove as fast as a race car driver. He wanted to get his new little niece into the arms of the pediatric specialists. They had been notified and were waiting with an incubator ready for the infant fighting for her life. As Don and Lily drove away with their precious passenger, Doc Smith and his nurse were watching—with no doubts in their minds—prayer, not medical care was now going to be their number one priority for this child. The medical odds were definitely not in the baby girl's favor.

∽

BILL WASN'T able to see Virginia for several days due to her being in quarantine and contagious, still fighting the virus and fever. The baby was handed over to a team of pediatric specialists at the teaching hospital. To avoid exposing the maternity ward to polio, quarantine was set up, and no one was allowed to see baby Dianne but the medical team. Although doctors did not diagnose the infant with polio, they knew that she had been exposed to her mother's polio, and that was enough to quarantine her.

So after the team finished examining and discussing the severity of baby Dianne's deformities, they diagnosed her with cerebral palsy. It had never been medically proven, or reported and published, that an infant could be polio in utero. None of them had ever seen a baby born from a polio-infected mother before. They didn't try to come up with a prognosis because none of them really believed the child would live long. They decided the family would have to wait until they all could agree upon one.

Virginia's fever broke on Wednesday night, which was almost three days from the time it began. Her legs were still very painful, but it wasn't as intense as days before. The medical team was not sure if the polio took her abilities to walk and move independently. She knew she was still very sick, but she wanted to see her baby girl and get home to her other babies. She was determined to get better. She was extremely weak when the nurses got her up to go to the bathroom, which of course didn't begin until after her fever broke. Everyone was thrilled that polio paralysis had not affected Virginia. However, she would have a long road of pain ahead of her before she could go home.

After Virginia's quarantine had been lifted, Bill drove over to the hospital to visit, and he filled her in on how Aunt Winnie (and Aunt Josie, Bill's Aunt, who lived two houses away and wanted to relieve Aunt Winnie occasionally), were taking care of Pat and Colleen. The children were fine, but they missed their mommy terribly. After all, they were so young and scared that their mom would never come back. Doc Smith received updates on baby Dianne's progress and care, but the news was not very hopeful from a medical standpoint. The specialized medical team was of a mind that the baby may still die, and even if she didn't, they felt certain she would never live a normal life. Doc Smith knew that kind of news was terrible for Virginia's recovery, so he just told Virginia and Bill that the baby was still in quarantine intensive care and that each day she lived was a good sign. Doc Smith had more to consider than just the prognosis of baby Dianne. He had to care for the entire family.

By the end of the first week after delivery, Virginia was able to get herself out of bed and to and from the bathroom without help. She worked hard to try and get her strength back in order to get home, though her pain was still in her limbs and back, and she certainly didn't have an appetite. However, she did accomplish her goal, and fourteen days after both giving birth and contracting polio, she was *released from the hospital. She was ordered by the doctors to be bedridden when she got home. Bill had to make sure there would be round-the-clock care at home waiting for Virginia, as well as for Pat and Colleen.*

Doc Smith came up and checked on Virginia every day for the following week. He also kept an eye on the rest of the family, since they were all exposed to the contagious polio virus. By the third week after the delivery, Virginia wanted to see her baby girl, but the doctors at the teaching hospital wouldn't allow it. Bill and Virginia were at the mercy of the medical experts. They didn't even know the names of the doctors who were treating their child. As county non-insured patients, they felt as if they had no rights to make demands or ask many questions. Bill knew that he only worked for the family business, and he knew he could not get insurance for himself and his family. His mother Lizzie never got employees coverage, and he was just that, an employee. So baby Dianne was a county patient at the very large teaching hospital, only qualified to be treated by a team of resident doctors just starting out. Bill knew that his child who was still fighting for her life needed the top-tier doctors that insurance companies paid for, but they were well out of his family's reach.

Finally, a month passed. Baby Dianne was still alive. Word came to Doc Smith that the parents could come down to see their baby. Virginia, though still weak, could hardly wait to see her. Bill was just plain scared. The drive was an hour-and-a-half away. They were both silent for most of the drive. They were both filled with questions that neither of them could answer. Not until they were with their child.

When they arrived at the teaching hospital, they checked in and waited to be called, like all the other people waiting. While they sat there, they noticed parents with their physically deformed children. Some were in wheelchairs. Some were able to walk but with braces, others with casts. Some of the children lay quietly in strollers, but were visibly different from physically normal-bodied infants and children. Bill and Virginia had no idea what they would see with their little girl. Doc Smith had only told them she was born paralyzed, with no physical description of the paralysis. They were told to expect her to be in an incubator for a while since she was born premature. That was the extent of what they knew.

A nurse finally called their names, "Mr. and Mrs. McTaggart," and they got up to follow her down the dreary, tan hallway with dingy, green linoleum. They were put into a room with curtains as dividers and told that the doctors would soon be in. It wasn't a long wait before two white-coat doctors entered, a woman and a man. The man spoke first, describing the treatment methods that were used to keep their infant alive. He said that IV's were still used to feed her and that she was still in the incubator, but she was breathing more on her own. They hoped that they could remove her from the incubator in a day or two. The doctor explained how they had diagnosed baby Dianne with the diagnosis of cerebral palsy, and not polio. Although they knew the baby had been born from a polio-stricken mother, they could not definitively say that the baby, too, had polio. In order to diagnose polio, the infant would have to have a spinal tap, the same test Doc Smith had prescribed for Virginia's diagnosis. It was the most definitive diagnostic tool doctors performed on patients suspected of contracting the polio virus. But they knew the baby was still in critical condition. If they did a spinal tap the baby would most likely die.

There was another reason why the doctors didn't diagnose baby Dianne with polio: None of them were aware of any reported case of polio in utero. Without published, empirical reports that polio in utero existed, the team of doctors used the best diagnosis they could. The doctor explained that every part of baby Dianne's body was paralyzed, except from her elbows to her hands. He also explained that children born with paralysis of this severity often didn't live long. He wanted to prepare them for what they were about to see. The female doctor didn't say anything and just deferred to the male doctor.

Bill and Virginia followed the doctors down the hall of the green linoleum, which they grew to hate. They entered a ward with incubators and cribs. They were taken to the incubator that held Dianne, their baby girl. What they saw was this tiny little baby with a bunch of tubes running all over and in her. Virginia clearly remembered seeing a beautiful head of black hair on her infant at the delivery, and yet her baby's head had been shaved due to the tubing needed to keep her alive. The doctor told them that she had gained a little weight and was up to about six pounds. That was a good sign. Virginia looked at her little girl, and she could see her baby's eyes looking around taking in all the activity. Virginia's heart wanted so much to pick her up and comfort her, but she knew she wouldn't be allowed to. Both she and Bill just watched their little one breathe and stay quiet in the little world the hospital had created for her.

Finally the female doctor spoke up and said, "As parents, you should be prepared to put this child in a home for crippled children. I do not feel the child will live long. I also believe that, even if the baby survives, she will never live a normal life. In my medical opinion, I have absolutely no doubt in my mind, the child will never be able to walk."

The male doctor broke into his colleague's speech, and he offered some reassuring words of hope. He ventured to say they were still not sure of the prognosis or lack of developmental progress the infant might have, but that if Bill and Virginia came back in a few days, they might know more.

As the doctors were preparing to take their leave, Virginia could not help but tell the female doctor, "Excuse me, doctor, but God did not give us this little girl just to put her away in some home for crippled children. I don't give a damn what your medical opinion is." The female doctor's face stayed stone-cold, and she did not respond. Virginia, looking at the male doctor's face, asked if she and Bill could stay a bit longer in the ward. He said for them to take their time, and the doctors would see them in a few days. Then the doctors turned away and left the room.

Virginia and Bill were both flooded with emotion as they stood looking at their baby girl. Each of them wanted to be strong for the other, so neither one cried. However, Virginia could not contain her anger toward the female doctor's statement, "Just admit your baby to the State home for crippled children!" Virginia was livid. How dare that doctor think that she and Bill could ever be so cold and heartless. How dare she call herself a doctor. Virginia named her the Grim Reaper.

Bill had to calm Virginia down. He too felt every bit of Virginia's anger, but that anger had to be put away. They were now facing the biggest challenge of their life together, and they didn't know how they would take care of their disabled child, but they knew they had to try.

∼

AND TRY THEY DID. Mom and Dad brought me home from the hospital about three-and-a-half months after I was born. I was still paralyzed from head to toe, but all the tubes and needles were out of me. Doctors had concluded that the paralysis did not affect the muscles of my mouth for swallowing or lungs for breathing. I was able to suck on a bottle and breathe completely on my own without the need for oxygen. (Everyone who knows me well today knows that I was definitely born with plenty of hot air.)

Mom told me that she cried when she first held me, because I was so frail. She told me that she was scared when she first picked me up, because she believed I could break. Mom clearly remembered how my legs and arms and head were so twisted when I was delivered, and my little head could not turn.

My legs were in a permanent frog-like position, and my arms were bent at the elbow and did not straighten, so she did not know how she could hold me without hurting me. However, a hospital nurse showed her how to wrap me up safely in a blanket.

All the nurses that had been my "hospital mothers" learned to adapt their normal infant care to a new, unique "Dianne care." So before sending me home, the nurses shared all their creative and caring tricks they had used, and that way, my parents could add them to the list of tricks and adaptive skills of their own. The nurses felt reassured knowing that I had steadily gained weight and was around eight pounds. I was making progress each day.

As the nurses said goodbye to me, they told my parents I was a born fighter. Mom and Dad happily left the hospital with me, and I finally arrived home.

Both of my grandmothers, as well as many aunts and uncles, were waiting at the house for our arrival. They all wanted to see the little baby they had been praying so hard for during the past three months. None of them were able to visit me in the hospital, since the doctors would not allow any visitors except for my parents. When Mom and Dad walked into the house with the newest member of the family, Aunt Winnie and Aunt Josie, who had taken turns babysitting Pat and Colleen since September, were there making sure that everyone was following the crowd-control rules.

My brother Pat told me years later that Mom and Dad told him and Colleen to treat their little sister "very special!" I learned that when I was preparing to write my story, and was asking him some questions of how much he remembered of the events of my birth. I wasn't sure what he remembered, being only four years old at the time. I only wish I had known that earlier. It would have been a perfect guilt-producing line, "to treat me special" — wow, I could have really gotten some mileage out of that one, throwing it at them every time they were doing their BIG BROTHER AND OLDER SISTER routines!

Anyway, I was a special attraction to all on that homecoming day, and I know heaven heard many prayers of thanksgiving from my family that night. In fact, Mom and Dad said that almost everyone in our little town gave out a huge sigh of relief when I arrived home.

Routines started to be established, with Mom taking care of the house and kids, and Dad going back to work. Dad had arranged for some of the family's older, girl cousins to take turns living with us. Dad knew that Mom needed babysitting help. Since Pat and Colleen were very active toddlers, Mom had to balance the special needs I required and still be a mom to Pat and Colleen.

Unfortunately, little Colleen, who was only 17 months older than me and a very quiet and shy child, felt invisible when family or neighbors stopped by. Everyone wanted to see the "special attraction." Pat, too, was affected by lack of attention and he learned to act out. He often picked on Colleen to make her scream and cry. His bad behaviors did get him attention but not the kind that was needed.

Mom and Dad did the best they knew how at the time. They created many routines that made things easier for the whole family. Mom always made everyone's beds every morning, and she had breakfast ready for the family by the time my dad left for work by eight o'clock. She cooked the family supper and had it ready everyday at half past five. No matter how exhausted she felt, or how weak her legs and arms were from the polio, she ran the house like clockwork.

However, some of those routines put Mom's own recovery on the back burner. Like most polio survivors, she pushed through it all and never gave in to her pain. She knew the pain, and where it came from, but decided that she would have a normal life as a wife and mother of three, in spite of it.

∼

My parents still made the hour-and-a-half drive down to the teaching hospital for my checkups once a month. We were still uninsured county patients, so checkups required waiting at least two to three hours before we were led into a curtained cubicle. Once there, we might have to wait yet another hour before the teaching doctor and his group of residents would enter.

None of the visits were the same. My parents never knew who the lead teaching doctor or resident doctors would be. They never got the same doctors twice.

I was being passed around to be studied by the orthopedic teaching department. Each time my parents left the hospital, they would leave knowing nothing more of a prognosis than when they came in. When my mother would tell the doctors— and there was always more than one doctor in the room—that I was eating and sleeping well, totally aware and engaged with the world and people around me, smiling and giggling at times, the doctors would just look blankly at her and nod. Dad and Mom felt like the doctors never heard a single word they spoke. They never showed any interest in the progress Mom described to them. How my parents kept their faith in doctoring was phenomenal. They never forgot what the original female doctor recommended to them about institutionalizing me, so they just kept trying to get doctors to listen to them. Many parents would have given up but for their belief that God wanted them to keep trying.

They were starting to grow weary and quite frustrated. They wanted answers and suggestions of what to do to help me progress, but doctors never gave them any hope or suggestions on home-based interventions that might help in my recovery. The family physician, Doc Smith, told my parents he did not feel qualified to advise them on my physical deformities, since he was just a family doctor. He always referred my parents to the teaching hospital doctors.

Mom decided that she had to get some medical advice from somewhere. So, she made an appointment with the town chiropractor. He explained how massage could increase the circulation in my little twisted body, and explained how, by increasing circulation, it would aid in healing. He also suggested using sandbags to try to straighten my frog-position legs. When Mom asked him if my legs would break if she tried to straighten them, it really showed how little guidance my parents were given by the orthopedic doctors.

The chiropractor listened patiently to my mom and was very helpful. He smiled reassuringly, and he proceeded to minimally manipulate my legs with much caution. He was testing and observing if the paralysis could be moved without causing me any pain. When he gently went to pull on my legs, he was amazed to see that I was ticklish. That told him that my paralyzed legs had feeling. In his experience, that was seldom seen in cases of paralysis. It was clear to him that a very small degree of straightening could be a possibility. However, he did not feel medically qualified to do the total manipulation, and he suggested my parents specifically ask the doctors at my next checkup. My mother just laughed at that suggestion and proceeded to describe the typical checkup to him. She told the chiropractor that talking to those doctors was like talking to a brick wall.

Thanks to the chiropractor's advice, Mom designed her own massage method for my tiny, contorted body. She used her favorite massage cream, cocoa butter, and began to massage and straighten my legs with sandbags each night. As the weeks passed, she and Dad saw very small signs of improvement. They wondered how they would explain my progress to a group of doctors who only studied my case file of symptoms, not me as a person.

My parents came to a decision—they had to try to find a doctor who would listen and work with them. The fighting spirit in me that was making progress kicked up the fighting spirits in them, too. So, my dad made a very fateful and fruitful telephone call—one that he had been thinking of making for quite some time.

My dad had a half-brother, Kenneth Brinkhous, who was born several years before my Grandma Lizzie married my Grandpa Michael McTaggart. Uncle Kenneth had graduated from medical school. Although he was now on the faculty of a university in another state, my dad knew Uncle Kenneth was still familiar with several doctors at the nearby teaching hospital. Dad decided to ask him for advice. What better network for advice could there be? Uncle Kenneth was a brilliant doctor, and later in his career, due to his voluminous research, he became the leading medical authority in hemophilia.

Grandma Lizzie's parents raised my Uncle Kenneth, so Dad was never as close with him as brothers can be. Plus, Dad was fourteen years younger than his brother Uncle Kenneth. However, Dad made the call, and Uncle Kenneth agreed to talk to his colleagues at the teaching hospital. Uncle Kenneth found out, through his inquiries with his medical school classmates, that there was a young orthopedic surgeon from Spain who was on staff at the teaching hospital's orthopedic department. He had arrived during the war in 1941.

According to my uncle's resources, this man, whose name was Dr. Ignacio Ponseti, came to the teaching hospital after escaping the Spanish Civil War. Dr. Ponseti used his orthopedic skills during his country's war, but he had to leave Spain and escape the war via Mexico, where he became a village doctor for a short time. All of Uncle Kenneth's medical contacts remarked on how Dr. Ponseti was a highly-respected physician and was known to have a wonderful, gentle way with children. Uncle Kenneth personally called Dr. Ponseti to ask if he would consider examining me and study my case. Thankfully, Dr. Ponseti graciously accepted.

That was the end of my parents' frustrations and the beginning of my wonderful medical care.

When I consider how my parents were uninsured and had very little money to spend on medical care, I shake my head at the huge gift Uncle Kenneth arranged. I can honestly say that the prayers of my family and townsfolk were really answered—especially on the day I became the patient of and placed into the medical hands of Dr. Ignacio Ponseti. Rarely does anyone find an orthopedic surgeon who is conservative when it comes to doing surgery. He really was. Dr. Ponseti was once interviewed by The Chicago Tribune in 2006 on being the innovator of a revolutionary treatment method for clubfoot. He was asked why it took so long for the orthopedic surgeons of the world to adopt his non-surgical treatment method, which he had developed years earlier while still in Spain. He replied, "Surgeons love their little knives."

Dr. Ponseti was my doctor for the first twenty-five years of my life with polio. He was my hero and medical angel. However, I am getting ahead of myself and my story, so let's get back to how I progressed.

~

MY MOTHER WAS my first physical therapist. She would put Pat and Colleen to bed each night and then keep me up to massage my limbs and sandbag my legs. After our therapy sessions, she would reward us with slices of garden-fresh tomatoes and pieces of cheddar cheese. She would get herself a cold bottle of beer, and then dip her finger in the beer to let me have a taste—but only one! Years later when I was in college, I would tell my mom about drinking beer at the college hangout. Mom would laugh and say, "It was all those good physical therapy sessions that led you to the beer, Honey."

When my mom showed Dr. Ponseti what the town chiropractor had taught her about massage and sandbagging, Dr. Ponseti agreed with that advice. He then taught my mother the proper way to do it. My parents were thrilled to finally have a doctor who gave them advice on my care. He gave them hope and assurances that they, as young parents, needed.

Years before I became his patient, Dr. Ponseti had designed the Ponseti Method of treating infants with clubfoot. It used casting the disabled foot, instead of performing surgery on the children. It was a non-invasive, non-surgical way of treating infants. The parents of those children afflicted with clubfoot truly welcomed the gentler treatment option for their child's physical defect.

Dr. Ponseti was a perfect teacher for my mother to learn from. He told my parents his plan to have them work with me at home to build up my strength. He then planned on casting my legs for about a month or two, in order to straighten them. Ultimately, he had to use the casting in intervals for over two years before I could straighten my legs on my own. Like I said before—he was a conservative surgeon. Historically, many polio children were victims of experimental surgeries. Knowing that history confirms my memory of just how blessed I was to have Dr. Ignacio Ponseti.

Dad once told me that Uncle Kenneth was very happy with Dr. Ponseti's conservative orthopedic treatment plan. Uncle Kenneth always said, "There is no such thing as minor surgery, since anesthesia is used in all surgeries and that makes all surgeries major." My parents were very happy to not face putting me through surgery and long hospital stays.

My speech and cognitive development was in the normal range for first-year babies. By the time I was seven or eight months old, I could be supported with pillows and bolsters to the sitting position on the sofa, but I could not sit up on my own. I had to be in the prone position most of the time due to extreme torso weakness.

The main carpet layer at my grandmother's furniture store was a very good carpenter. He took a wooden infant highchair, and sawed off some sections and sanded them down so that my frog legs could fit in the chair. My parents were then able to securely strap me in place, and I finally sat at the dinner table with my whole family.

The carpenter's name was Steny. He was a wonderful man and a true friend to my parents. He and his wife Marie were from Poland. They were WWII survivors, as well as survivors of a displaced person's camp. My family sponsored them when they immigrated to America, along with their young son who was born in the camp. They wanted to come to America after they were liberated from the Nazi regime. Steny had a huge heart and a very "can-do" spirit. Mom and Dad built their family around the challenges that came with my disability, and with friends like Steny who gave his creative adaptive skills abundantly, I experienced a very loving, independent environment.

I believe having so much extended family within blocks of each other made it possible for my parents to live life with extra support. Money was really tight, but love was plentiful and accessible for the asking. Both of my parents told me how their faith was their anchor. I don't think it was an accident that they met at St. Joseph's Catholic School while in junior high (now known as middle school). The small town of Elkader, with a population of barely one thousand, was the type of setting where neighbors and friends were always there to help. St. Joseph's parishioners were the center source of prayer and hope. The priest and nuns always kept my entire family in their daily prayers. And thank God they were, because little did my parents know, that they were about to be hit yet again with another medical roller coaster ride. It was in the fall of 1954, about a year after my birth.

Virginia was so tired of trudging up and down the sixteen steps several times a day just to get to the four bedrooms, but somebody had to make the beds and clean upstairs. She was also exhausted when she had the laundry to do down in the basement, which was another thirteen steps down and back up to the kitchen. She knew that her legs were weaker after the polio, which was only a year ago. Stairs were a part of life in their home, so she just kept plugging away. Aunt Winnie and Aunt Josie took turns helping Virginia out during the day with taking care of the three kids. Pat was an active four-going on five-year-old, but he was still not old enough to be in school. Little Colleen was only two-and-a-half and still in need of attention and care. Dianne was still paralyzed and needed to be held or positioned safely in her crib or on the changing table that had been set up in the kitchen so Virginia could keep an eye on her while she was cooking or doing dishes.

Bill was putting in as many hours as possible down at the store, but Lizzie didn't increase his salary no matter how many hours he worked. He had noticed that he was losing weight and was always exhausted. He told himself that he should feel that way working and coming home and helping with the kids. Life was exactly as they could expect in their situation, so Bill, like Virginia, pushed on.

One day, as Bill was getting ready for work, he noticed a hard lump along the side of his neck while in the shower. He didn't remember feeling that before, so he thought he'd keep an eye on it to see if it would go away on its own. He knew he had too much to do to worry about a lump. Virginia and he had just taken Dianne to the teaching hospital the previous week. Dr. Ponseti had put Dianne in her first casts, one for each leg. The doctor was hoping it could be the beginning of straightening her frog legged position, and both he and Virginia prayed for it to work. Pat and Colleen got to color some flowers on Dianne's casts. The two older children had learned to accept many different things during the past year, so coloring on their baby sister's casts was part of their normal life together.

The first casts were only on for a month, but little Dianne was happy to get them off. Her legs were straight when the casts were removed, but they had to be sandbagged many times during the day to stay straight. Progress was being made slowly, and Bill knew God was still answering prayers like always.

Doc Smith wanted to keep up with Dianne's progress as well, so one day Bill took Dianne down to his office for a checkup. While he was there, Doc Smith asked Bill how he was feeling, since the Doc saw how thin and tired he looked. Bill was honest with him and told him how beat he really was.

Bill mentioned the lump he had found on his neck several weeks ago. Doc Smith felt it, and then he felt under Bill's arms. He told Bill that it concerned him. Since the teaching hospital was so familiar to the family, Doc Smith called them while Bill was still in the office and made an appointment for Bill to see a surgeon there. He explained to Bill that it could be many things, but a biopsy had to be done to diagnose the lump. He also told Bill that it could be cancerous, so he and Virginia had to act on it right away.

Just what Bill wanted to hear, another trip to the hospital. Cancer wasn't in Bill and Virginia's plans at all. It had never entered their minds before. Bill told Virginia his news that night, once the kids were in bed. Virginia was sure it was not cancer, but she was so happy that Doc Smith had made the appointment for that same week.

They lined up Aunt Josie to watch the kids, and the two of them drove the hour-and-a-half drive down to the teaching hospital. It had once been a place they thought once only as the home of a state football team and the college Bill attended for a year before he had to go off and do his duty as a soldier in WWII. Now the teaching hospital had become almost a home-away-from- home for Dianne's care.

Bill and Virginia knew they needed another miracle if the lump was cancerous. They drove to the place they put so much time and trust in during the past year—where they now prayed a miracle might happen again. They believed this to be true. For the teaching hospital gave them Dianne, a living miracle.

The biopsy went as planned, and they were able to come home that same night. Bill knew it would be a while before they got the biopsy results, but he and Virginia were glad that the results would be sent to Doc Smith, so they didn't have to drive back down to the hospital again. Family life and work went on as normal. About three days after the biopsy, Doc Smith phoned and asked if he could come up to the house to talk. Both Virginia and Bill had a sick feeling, but they scheduled the Doc to come over right after supper. He arrived on time and didn't beat around the bush.

He told them that the lump was malignant, but that he didn't know what the prognosis was. He explained that it could be a form of cancer called Hodgkin's Disease, but only the teaching hospital doctors would know for sure. Doc Smith had set up another appointment for Bill to visit the medical team so they could explain the next step in treatment. Doc Smith told them he was sorry he had bad news to deliver, but he felt they were in good hands with the teaching hospital. He saw his own way out that night so Bill and Virginia could talk privately.

∼

As Bill and Virginia looked at each other, they both wanted a good stiff drink. Pat and Colleen were fighting, and Dianne was in Virginia's lap, so there was no time for those drinks. They got the kids ready for bed, and Virginia decided to skip Dianne's physical therapy that night. They put all three kids to bed at the same time. They needed their private time.

Bill and Virginia were scared, and both of them knew it. Being strong for each other was really getting old. They shared their fears and then their prayers. Afterward, they were so tired, they decided to go to bed early that night, but neither slept very well.

Bill was thinking about his family and how in the world could Virginia handle all this without him. Virginia lay awake thinking about how her mother Ella became a widow with three kids just a month after Virginia had been born. She knew how hard life was for her mom and how they all struggled to make ends meet. Ella took in boarders to keep a roof over their heads after she lost the family farm due to her husband's death. Virginia wondered if she would be like her mother, a struggling widow with three kids.

Sleep was not in the cards for her that night, but she decided to pray as she lay there in bed. She believed that somehow God would answer her prayers. Bill prayed silently too, as he tried to get some sleep knowing he had to be up early for work. Tomorrow would come soon enough, and in a few days so would another trip to the teaching hospital.

Their hospital trip was upon them before they knew it, and Aunt Winnie was scheduled to watch Pat, Colleen, and Dianne. Aunt Winnie knew what they were facing, since Virginia confided in her. Like her sister Ella, Aunt Winnie used the family's favorite mantra, "God is Good." Virginia grew up hearing that from her mother on a daily basis, so she decided to hang on to that thought while they drove to the hospital.

The two of them arrived and checked in. After an hour's wait, a nurse came to get them. Bill and Virginia both remembered the last time a nurse at that same hospital came to take them to a roomful of doctors. It had only been a year ago when they met the first team of doctors who gave them their prognosis for Dianne. Now it was a new team of doctors with another prognosis, but this time it was for Bill. This prognosis, like the last one, could change their family life in an instant.

Bill and Virginia went in and sat down at a table, where seven doctors were waiting. Two doctors were sitting at the conference table, with two chairs waiting for Bill and Virginia. The five student residents stood along the wall behind the two lead doctors. The room was so small, that Bill and Virginia felt like they were in a cell—a cell with the detestable green linoleum floor. The lead doctor explained the biopsy findings and said, "Mr. McTaggart, you have a very advanced case of Hodgkin's Disease, and we are very sorry to tell you and your wife this, but the prognosis is not good. It is our opinion that you have less than a year to live." At that point Bill turned white. Virginia sat silent staring down at a sea of green linoleum and feeling like she was seasick. She snapped out of her daze and looked at Bill. She asked the doctors if she and Bill could go outside in the hall to talk for a minute. The doctors thought that was a good idea, so they left the room.

Numb was not even close to what Bill felt, and tears welled up in his eyes as he looked at Virginia. He didn't know what to say to her. Virginia knew Bill very well, and so she took his hand and said, "Now Bill, we have to face this together, and this is what I think: You don't have time to die Bill! You and I both know God did not give us our three kids just to have you die, so we have to go back in that room and tell those doctors to do everything medically possible to get you through this. Okay?" They both had tears in their eyes, but they each took a deep breath, wiped their tears away, and went into that room once more with the fighting spirit they were both born with. Bill told the doctors, "Whatever treatment you have, I want to try." They explained that cobalt therapy was grueling and risky, plus they could not guarantee the outcome. Virginia looked re-assuredly at Bill while *holding his hand, as Bill looked away. He centered his eyes on the two sitting doctors and said, "Do whatever it takes."*

~

MY DAD WENT through the cancer treatment with lots of help from the Elkader community. The businessmen of Main Street and even the parish priest took turns driving Dad to and from the hospital for weekly cobalt radiation treatments. Years later, my dad told me the radiation technicians had to draw on his body with permanent black marker, in order to know where the radiation beams would go that day. He had to lay still on a hard X-ray table for hours, as his Elkader drivers patiently waited for him in the waiting room. My dad said that he never wanted to smell the ink of a black marker again for as long as he lived. Since I was only two years of age at the time, I only know that my parents made it through by the grace of God and being surrounded with loving support of family and friends. Dad beat the odds and pulled through all the cancer treatments. The nuns and priest had another miracle to thank God for. Mom was right—Dad did not have time to die.

~

IN EARLY 1957, when I was about three-and-a-half years old, I started to develop enough strength in my torso to sit up in a chair for short periods of time on my own. I no longer needed to have someone support me or be strapped into the chair in order to sit up. Steny had built a specially designed balance-bar walking area for me to hang onto. Each side had a soldered steel handlebar to grip. It was about five to six feet long, and wide enough for my twenty-pound body to support itself with mom's help, as I grabbed ahold of each side bar. Steny's design was perfect. It even included a glued rubberized floor so that my leather-soled orthopedic shoes would not slip. Dad had positioned a full-length mirror near one end so I could see myself walking.

Even with all the trials my parents had gone through in the past three and a half years, God decided to bless them with another child. A baby boy was born in January 1957. They named him Kevin. You can imagine how scared they both were having another child after the experience of my delivery. Doc Smith kept a careful eye on Mom's pregnancy, watching for any effects that her polio infection might cause. However, the delivery went smoothly and Kevin was a very healthy, happy baby. I became a big sister now, no longer the baby of the family. Kevin and I became quite a pair. I loved all my siblings, but Kevin and I had what I call a "magical" connection. We both liked getting into trouble together, and I liked it most of all because Kevin was the one who always got caught.

Pat and Colleen had started school and I was still doctoring at the teaching hospital every two to three months. Mom was faithful with my home physical therapy program that she and Dad had developed. Dr. Ponseti was very pleased with my progress. Aunt Winnie or Aunt Josie took turns being the family babysitter for Kevin. They always helped Mom with the housework and all the chores that motherhood creates. Mom and I worked hard on my therapy program every day while Pat and Colleen were in school and Dad was at work. One day, when I was a few months shy of my fourth birthday, I took my very first step without the balance-bar handles. Of course, my mom was "over the moon" with excitement, but she wanted to make sure I could really walk before she told anyone, even Dad. She told me it would be our secret.

As a few days went by, my mom knew I was sufficiently stable and sure-footed to reveal our secret. I still remember the evening when Dad came home from work. Mom, who always had supper ready, told Dad, Pat and Colleen to sit down in the living room. She said, "Dianne has to show you all something." Kevin was in his playpen happily playing with his toys. Mom had me sitting in a chair before Dad came home, and I kept our secret from Pat and Colleen like my mother told me to. Once I had all their attention, Mom told me to go ahead and share our secret. My chair was positioned closest to Dad. I got up with mom's help, and she let go of me. I had my eyes on Dad, and then took my first independent steps straight into his arms. His face had the biggest smile on it while he hugged me as I came up to him. Pat and Colleen wanted me to walk to them too, which I did. From that night on, there was no stopping me. Some things I have never forgotten, and that is surely one of my happiest memories. I also remember them clapping for me, which I believe marks the day I was bitten by the bug to become an entertainer!

Word of my walking spread fast in our little town. The priest and nuns declared that God had worked another miracle. Not only did I live when the doctors said I probably wouldn't, but now I walked though doctors were positive I never would. I should clarify, that there was one doctor who believed I would do this, that I could eventually walk—Dr. Ponseti. He was "somebody who told me I could."

My family also believed that I could eventually walk and do many other things that doctors could not medically explain. I was ready for more challenges. I was dreaming of all the things I could do by myself, and even get into some trouble. . . all by myself!

When my parents took me to my next appointment with Dr. Ponseti, I wanted to walk into the examining room right away, but we had to wait our turn as we always did. It was a very long two to three-hour wait for me, being as excited as I was to share my new secret. My dad carried me into the draped cubicle as he always did. I saw the many resident student doctors looking at me, but my eyes were on Dr. Ponseti. When he asked how I was doing, Mom said, "Dianne, why don't you show Dr. Ponseti how you are doing?" Dad put me down and I stood by myself and looked straight at the doctor, glancing once over to the group of residents standing around. Dr. Ponseti was smiling widely, and his eyes sparkled as he saw me standing there. I then proceeded to walk on my own power straight into Dr. Ponseti's arms. He caught me in a big hug, and said, "Oh, My Dianne. How wonderful today is."

I remember him asking me to walk over to the residents, and I looked at him as if to say, "Are you kidding me?" He picked up on my look and immediately told me to just walk back to my parents and once more to him.

Although Dr. Ponseti always examined my physical abilities and strengths/weaknesses while lecturing and demonstrating to his students, today he didn't do a physical exam. He just lectured the residents on how I was his puzzle child, and that they should learn that what they might read in a file is not always easily explained, nor is it always accurate. I now look back and marvel on Dr. Ponseti's style of teaching and how he always made me feel safe. For being such a young child, I felt safe and protected by this doctor in a huge hospital, and that speaks volumes about how blessed I was to receive such high-quality medical care by such a special doctor. He always called me "My Dianne" whenever I came for my appointments, and I still hear his voice calling me his Dianne to this very day. No wonder I always felt safe.

PART II
THE SCHOOL YEARS

2

Since I was examined, studied and discussed each time I went to the teaching hospital, the discussion among the young doctors and the senior ones like Dr. Ponseti, would get around to my diagnosis of being born with polio. As I explained earlier, I was originally diagnosed as a cerebral palsy patient since polio in utero had never been medically reported in any journals.

Around the age of four, Dr. Ponseti had me tested by a speech pathologist. I remember my mom accompanied me into the examining room as the pathologist directed me to sit in a child-size chair on the far side of the room. She asked me if I could answer her questions, and I said yes. After a few questions, she asked if I would take a sucker and show her how I would eat it. I remember she asked me what flavor I'd like, and I said strawberry. She then watched as I sucked the sucker. She just watched me and wrote things down in her notebook, never speaking to me or my mom. I looked across the room at my mom, with a look on my face that said, "This is stupid." I wanted to stop.

Mom read my face and told me I should be a good girl. "Just

do as the nice lady says." I looked over to the pathologist as she stared at me. I paused thinking this really WAS stupid, so I threw the sucker across the room. It shattered all over the floor. The pathologist looked up and laughed saying, "Well there's nothing wrong with your mouth or facial muscles, Dianne." She then looked over to my mom and said, "I don't see any problem with your daughter's speech and language development, possible indicators of cerebral palsy. In my opinion, that diagnosis is wrong. I am documenting my findings in her file for the rest of the medical team to consider." Dr. Ponseti took her recommendation and noted polio was the cause of my disability. Young residents never won any argument with Dr. Ponseti from that point forward.

By the age of five, I still couldn't walk up and down stairs, but I could crawl up and scoot down the steps to my bedroom. I got stronger each year, but was not physically up to starting kindergarten at age five. The public school had kindergarten, but all of their playground areas were covered with gravel, which was totally dangerous and non-accessible for me. I only weighed about 25 pounds, and if a strong wind came up, down I'd go.

Falling was everyday normal to me. Other than skinned knees and shins, I was pretty tough. I figured ways of getting myself up from most falls, since I wasn't very far from the ground even standing. With my torso muscles so weakened by polio, I had developed a severe scoliosis which made my left leg about two and a half inches shorter than my right, but I adapted my gait to walking on my left toes. Mom told me I was practicing to be a ballerina. To this day, my left heel is as round and soft as an infant's foot.

I began school as a first grader when I was 6, skipping kindergarten. The year was 1959. I went to the parochial school at St. Joseph's Parish. I still couldn't climb stairs, and the first-grade classroom was up two big flights, plus three steps to get into the school. The worst part of all was that bathrooms were down another two flights of stairs to the basement.

The principal, who was one of the several nuns who taught at the school, was my first teacher. She taught me for first and second grade. All classrooms had two grades in one room at St. Joseph's Parochial School, better known as St. Joe's. Sister designed a program to assign a rotating list of eighth-grade boys to be my transportation up and down the stairs. Sister also hoisted me up and down steps a great deal of the time too. As to my personal hygiene needs, I learned to "hold it" until lunchtime and even held it until I got home from school at 3:30.

I remember hating being carried everywhere. Some kids were cruel and laughed, but Mom and Dad told me I had to be strong and thankful for all the help. I even developed a crush on one or two of the boys who I thought were cute and nice to me. I always felt very protected, and I thought my first teacher was the most wonderful teacher in the world. She became my first Americans with Disabilities Act (ADA) advocate, long before the ADA was ever thought of.

However, school was challenging my immunities and I developed pneumonia by November that first year at St. Joe's. I had to be hospitalized in the small, nearby hospital where I was born. Elkader still did not have a hospital yet. It was the first time I could remember being away from my parents, and I did not like the hospital. It was Thanksgiving week when I got sick, and I had to be in a children's ward. We were all in crib style beds, and sick kids are no fun to be around. My mom would visit every day, but hospitals were very strict about visitation hours, even for parents visiting their children.

My memories of my first hospitalization are not my happiest ones, but I sure remember the baby bed, the crying kids, and the medicine that was distributed in either apple sauce or egg nog. I still hate both of them today. However, I do have two nice memories of that time. The first one was that I made friends with the girl next to me. We both were small enough to reach through the crib bars and share our dolls with each other which really helped pass our days faster. The second memory was that my friend and I got to go home at the same time. After a week in the hospital, I was more than ready to get sprung, and she was too!

However, my body was still too weak to go back to school that year. I had to start first grade again the following year when I was seven years old. Of course, I tell everyone now that I flunked first grade. As I explained earlier, each classroom at St. Joe's school had two grades. When I made my first attempt at first grade, my sister Colleen was in second grade, so we were in the same classroom every day.

When I had to start all over again the following year, Colleen was in the third grade and in the classroom across the hall. It was hard for me to be in a brand-new class and yet have my old first-grade classmates in the same room. They got to move up a grade, and I didn't. I did get teased about not being smart enough to keep up with them, but I learned that my new first-grade classmates were lots more fun. Looking back now, I know I was always supposed to be with that class. As for the teasing, I had a mouth on me, which I still do, and learned how to stick up for myself with no problem. Well, not much of a problem except when the nuns *overheard* some comments, and then I would put on a big smile for them, and use my best limp while turning away. Usually worked too!

As I explained earlier, I was in the new first-grade class and my sister Colleen went up to third grade. We were in different classrooms now, and we both realized we liked that. I couldn't tell on her, and she couldn't tell on me. Sisters will be sisters. And speaking of sisters, the year 1960 brought us both a new little sister, Maureen. She was so anxious to come into the world, she was born in the front seat of the family station wagon while

Dad was driving Mom to the closest hospital, in a neighboring town, since Elkader still did not have its own hospital yet, even in 1960. Doc Smith was following in his car about ten minutes behind them. Dad had to pull off the highway and deliver his new little McTaggart girl, with Mom talking, or should I say, screaming him through it. Thank God Doc Smith knew their car by sight, because he pulled up behind them just in time to cut the umbilical cord. When Dad later told the story of Maureen's birth, he said he was so relieved to see Doc Smith, because he knew he would have fainted cutting the chord. Mom and Dad now had five kids. Like I said at the beginning of my story, God had different plans than that young McTaggart couple.

~

It was 1962, and I was eight years old finishing second grade. I could take one stair step at a time very slowly with my right leg, which I called my "good" leg. Sister allowed me to try a few times, but most of the time I was still carried up and down by the eighth graders. It got to the point where I hated being treated like a baby. So over the summer between second and third grade, I practiced my stair-stepping at home every day. My speed got better, but I could never use my left leg to step up or down. It was my right leg only, and it still is the stronger leg. Polio survivors often refer to their "good" leg or arm. Polio never struck any survivor the same way, so not everyone with polio had a good limb, but many did. In reality though, today's post-polio specialists, physiatrists, have explained to polio survivors that all of our limbs were affected by the polio strike, but the degree of weakness that develops varies in each one of us as we age.

St. Joseph's Parochial School, grades first through eighth, had maybe 100 students total at any one time. It was a very old building, built in 1911, and I knew every creaky step in the place. I did master all of those steps by the time I turned ten years old. I even made it down to the basement restrooms. The basement also had a little room for an infirmary and two rooms for private music lessons.

When I was in fourth grade, I began taking piano lessons, since I was able to maneuver all the way to and from the basement on my own. The lessons were taught by one of the nuns. I tried to take lessons earlier, when I was 8 years old and in the second grade. However, my arms were too weak, and I had a hard time reaching the piano. Plus, I still had to be carried up and down the steps.

When I finally began my piano lessons, neither the teacher nor my parents expected me to be a virtuoso pianist, but they thought it would be good exercise for my arms. I know that was the beginning of my love for music therapy, though my parents didn't call it that. I loved music so much that making all those steps for the lessons, as well as the practice times during the week, didn't bother me. St. Joe's was definitely not accessible, but I adapted and grew stronger each year. There were many steps to conquer. All students attended daily 11:30 Mass in the church, which had about eight steps to enter, and then we walked over to the lunchroom hall which had four steps to enter.

Iowa weather wasn't easy on me. Iowa winters produced ice and snow that could begin as early as October and extend all the way to mid-April. It was not unusual for the entire month of January to be 30° below zero. The severe weather shifts that occurred year-round produced many days of high winds. I never had enough strength to keep my balance in very high winds. Windy days meant falling to me. However, on those windy days Sister's buddy system kicked in, so I always had another student designated to help me when I needed help. Sometimes that meant hanging onto me in the wind, keeping me down to earth!

I really related to a popular television show about a light-weight nun who couldn't keep her feet on the ground during windy days. As far as ice and snow obstacles, the buddy system helped with that too. Long before the ADA was law, Sister was my advocate.

My falls were unfortunately frequent, and I would go down very quickly. My parents called me their rag doll because of the way I would just plop. Little did I know growing up that I could have made some serious money as a stunt woman. I could have taught stunt people how to fall and not get hurt...well, not much!

That buddy system was sewn into the fabric of my whole parochial education. At recess, the nuns had us play softball, so my classmates volunteered to be my runner when I would have a chance at bat. I was also a pretty good pitcher with my left arm. I experienced what it was like being on a softball team thanks to that buddy system. Even later, in seventh and eighth grades, when girls' softball teams would be formed to compete with the neighboring towns' Catholic schools, I was the official score keeper and cheer leader for my team. I had recess "buddies" who would help me swing on the large swing-set. They would stand on the swing seat pumping me up high in the air, while I sat on the seat. I felt such a thrill and loved going higher and higher. My friends included me in everything. I even had a pair of roller skates like the other girls. Our teacher would let us bring them from home to use at recess. Obviously I couldn't roller skate like other kids. My body could never do that. However, two of my friends would each take one of my arms and help me up after I put the skates on, and off the three of us went. In my head, I could skate and play ball and do whatever the other kids did, thanks to Sister's buddy system, and...... because "somebody told me I could."

Although I was doing fine in parochial school, my disability still had to be monitored at the teaching hospital every 6 months with Dr. Ponseti, with his students studying my case. The routine was always the same. I would be placed in the small, draped examining cubicle and handed a "stylish" hospital gown that was ALWAYS huge on me. I then had to undress down to my underwear and socks and put on their ugly gown. I would then wait for Dr. Ponseti and his students to enter.

That routine was a condition of my being treated as an uninsured patient at the teaching hospital. All county patients, meaning uninsured patients, were required to check in by 8:00 a.m. My parents were always at my side, and we would leave our house around six o'clock in the morning to check in by the hospital's required time. We were usually called after a two to three-hour wait, and then we were led into the partitioned, curtained room that was never bigger than ten feet by ten feet. Dr. Ponseti would enter and go over to his chair with his students all around him. He would greet me with the warmest smile, and I would always hear his gentle voice say, "Ah, My Dianne." He would look up at the six to seven medical students, standing around his chair waiting for his instruction and say, "She is my puzzle child."

He would begin his examination of me by pointing out to each batch of new students what I could and could not do. Dr. Ponseti would then tell the students that my file would not explain what they were about to see me do. He would have me bend over and trace my spine, checking my scoliosis. He had me walk back and forth repeatedly, which wasn't easy to do in such a tiny space. The students would watch. He would tell his students that medically I should not be able to walk as I did. He explained that my muscles didn't receive messages from my brain in order to contract or expand.

He would ask them what they thought, and a lively discussion ensued. Dr. Ponseti directed his students to ask me questions, like, "Can you raise your arms?" I would always reply, "I can't." Of course, Dr. Ponseti knew I could never raise my arms any higher than my waist. My shoulder deltoid muscles were never functional due to the polio virus destroying the motor neurons. Essential motor neurons are needed to develop muscles to respond. Many muscles throughout my body did not have motor neurons attached to them.

Dr. Ponseti would smile, looking at me and say, "Dianne, show the students how you brush your hair. Then show them how you wash your hair, or reach for something in a kitchen cupboard." He had me demonstrate the medical puzzle I presented to any team of doctors. I listened to them discuss me in a language I didn't understand (better known as medical jargon to me), and the examination/teaching session would wind down. It usually lasted thirty to forty-five minutes, ending around lunchtime. Dr. Ponseti would then tell my parents to take me to the X-ray department next, after we had gotten our lunch. I was always happy to put my own clothes back on again and have lunch.

The X-ray department was in another building on the hospital campus. I hated that the most. Dr. Ponseti requested images of my entire body, from head to toe, and in many different positions. Back in the 1950's and early 1960's, X-ray radiation levels were high for patients. The technicians were professionals I learned to respect. I listened to their explanations when they positioned my body while telling me what they were going to do next. They always gave the order, "Please hold still and do not breathe." I think that ultimately helped my vocal ability! I had to lie perfectly still for many hours on the table. I learned to hold my breath when the technician would go behind a partition with a glass window. X-ray imaging could take up to two hours.

Mom was always there to prepare me for the X-ray taking. I

would have to undress again and only be in my undershirt and underpants. Then Mom would leave the room. She always took the rest of my clothes and waited in an adjacent room. I was led by a stranger down the hall to the imaging area. X-ray technicians were mostly men in those days, and that was not fun for me, being a little girl who could only wear her underwear while they took X-rays. However, most of the technicians were pleasant and respectful of my feelings.

The long X-ray table was cold, black and very hard. Hospitals were and still are very cold, and blankets would interfere with the X-ray image. As I mentioned before, I learned early on to stay perfectly still and hold my breath. I learned that if I moved or breathed, I would have to be there longer, and I would be frozen to the bone. By the time I was around eleven, I could get up on the table by myself. However, before that age I experienced many years of strangers picking me up and positioning me onto that dreaded table. I later named the table *"the black icicle."*

Hours later, after the films were taken, my parents and I went back to Dr. Ponseti in the original building we had started the day in. Again, we waited at least an hour, maybe more. It took time for the X-ray images to be developed and delivered to Dr. Ponseti. We were finally called back into yet another curtained room. Dr. Ponseti would be standing and pointing to the illuminated X-rays on screens. He showed them to an even larger group of resident student doctors than he had taught earlier. He used me, and the X-rays of my body, as his teaching tools. The student doctors would look at me, then back to the X-rays of me, over and over again. Dr. Ponseti always told me that my spinal curve, scoliosis, could straighten itself by my body's movement. He had me demonstrate how I could easily move around in different positions that allowed my spine to nearly straighten itself without causing me any pain. The scoliosis was a three-area spinal curve: Cervical (neck), which was about a thirty percent curve; thoracic (lungs), which was about a forty-five percent curve; and lumbar (lower back). which was about a forty percent curve. Dr. Ponseti was happy that it stabilized by the time I was eight years old, but it was medically labeled as severe scoliosis.

There were always lots of questions posed to Dr. Ponseti from his students regarding my scoliosis. After all, this was an orthopedic department, and surgery was always a favorite topic. Young residents would argue for spinal fusion or Harrington Rod surgery, as well as shoulder fusion surgery for my left shoulder that was in partial subluxation, which is when a shoulder joint ball is not quite in the socket. Dr. Ponseti was always my advocate for disallowing invasive fixes for things that weren't really broken. I know now how rare it was to find a surgeon who thought that way. He always told me, "You will get along just fine Dianne." He was one of the most influential voices I heard who told me "I could." I always believed him, and I have lived my life with that belief.

I did need to have surgery when I was six years old. It was done to lengthen my left ankle, to see if it could catch up with my longer, right leg. I remember that well, and the cast I wore for three months during June through August. Talk about hot and itchy! However, that surgery didn't work. All I got from it was a three-inch ankle scar and a summer I couldn't swim. I think not being able to swim was my biggest complaint that summer. I don't remember the pain, though you can't have orthopedic surgery without it. Being in a cast and a wheelchair when I was so tiny wasn't that hard for rehab. I was small enough to have a full-time babysitter help Mom and Dad carry me around the house and up to bed and of course, to and from the toilet.

There was one other surgery I needed when I was twelve,

between sixth and seventh grades. Dr. Ponseti wanted to stunt the growth in my right leg before my final puberty growth spurt occurred. It required surgeons to dig the growth plate out of the bone below and around my knee. I didn't know that at the time but was told only that surgery had to be done then, before puberty set in. I was in the hospital for a week with another cast as before, from my toes to my hip. That surgery was extremely painful and I was in a children's ward at the end of July 1966. The temperature in Iowa was extremely hot and humid. Days of ninety degrees on up were normal, and the ward had no air conditioning, just pedestal fans.

I remember being scared and in pain, and they couldn't stop the bleeding after days following surgery. The wound bled through my thick cast. The red blood gradually dried to brown, and the person who made the cast later wrapped more casting plaster gauze around my knee so the cast could hold for the next six weeks. Mom visited me almost every day, and I made some friends on the ward with the other girls that also had orthopedic surgeries. I don't ever remember liking the nurses or many of the residents and other doctors that studied my case. However, when Dr. Ponseti would come in, I always felt like it was a visit from family, so I was okay.

When I was released to go home, the rehab required a hospital bed to be set up in the living room where the piano was. I was blessed with a terrifically strong, young babysitter named Sherry, who helped me in and out of bed and helped me with my toileting and sponge baths since I could not get the cast wet.

I got through all of that surgery and rehab intact, with lots of help and love from my parents and family and my sweet friend and babysitter Sherry. They all helped me stay occupied enough so I didn't get too bored in the wheelchair. I also figured out a neat trick with a wire coat hanger, that I used to stick down or up my cast to scratch the itch. In hindsight, I think that was pretty stupid, but at the time it was a brilliant relief. I was still mad that my summer swimming time was cut short by at least six weeks. To this day, I remember July 29, 1966. It was the last full day of swimming Mom let me have, and I stayed the whole day until the community pool closed at 9:00 p.m.. My surgery was set for July 30.

One of my fondest, and naughtiest, memories of time sitting in my wheelchair on our front porch was with my little sister Maureen, who was only five years old at the time. She was by my side a lot that summer wanting to play dolls and just help her big sister feel better. Well...we were outside, and I was bored to tears. I spotted one of our Uncle Don's cigarette butts just off the edge of the porch in the bushes. I told Maureen to go get it. She did whatever I told her to do, of course. Then I told her to go inside the house and go to the drawer in the kitchen where Mom kept the books of matches and bring one to me. I told her it was going to be our special secret. She went in and came out with a book of matches, and then I looked around to make sure nobody was around us, and I lit up the cigarette like a real hotshot, puffing away without even coughing—which was of course, not knowing how to inhale. Then Maureen begged to try it, too. Like a true friend, sister, and dumb twelve year old, I let her try a couple puffs. Fortunately, the butt was very short and stubby, and I swore Maureen to secrecy with a pinkie swear. We threw it over the porch after smashing it on a plate I had on my tray. To this day, we still both giggle at that, and she reminds me of how much of a *spectacular* influence I was on her growing up!

Maureen has also told me that she learned patience from me, since I had to sit and be at the mercy of others to help me do something. I could never wheel my own wheelchair, since my arms didn't, and still don't, have enough strength to move the wheels. My elementary school days of having to be carried around school served as a perfect foundation of patience and trust.

I developed trust early on with all my nurses, eighth-grade boys, babysitters and even strangers I'd occasionally need to pick me up off the ground when I would fall. I had to trust they wouldn't drop me. I developed patience with being a county uninsured patient at the teaching hospital with the all too common two to three-hour wait at my appointments.

I wish I could always tap into those life skills I learned at an early age when I get short-tempered and impatient now as an adult. I guess we all have early life skills we would do well to remember later on in life.

~

I WENT through my first eight years of schooling at St. Joe's with the same twelve kids in my class. I remember each student vividly, and I have many fond memories. However, there were a few memories that helped shape my outlook on life, although they weren't pleasant.

Think back with me to the surgery I had between sixth and seventh grade. It was a pretty big medical procedure and quite painful. I had the cast on for about six weeks, and then I had to get back to school. I couldn't bend my leg due to being in a cast for a solid block of time, so I learned ways to protect it. After the surgery, Dr. Ponseti told me that if I fell on the knee that had the surgery during the first six months to a year afterwards, I would have to go into surgery again.

Falling was something that was just another part of living for me. My falls could never really be predicted. But I certainly knew if I went over my limits of strength, I could easily fall. I also knew I had to dig deep down inside myself to be ultra-protective and aware of my surroundings. My classmates and seventh-grade teacher, who was also the principal of the school that year, were all told of my surgery and how serious my recovery was. My teacher, who was a new nun I had not had before, explained how they would all work together keeping me safe and protect me from falling. Well...all but one classmate.

He was the scrapper of the class and the biggest boy of all. Our desks were old wooden row desks, and my desk was often close to his. One afternoon, not long after I had returned to school from my surgery, I had to turn in a paper. I passed the scrapper's desk as I went to the front of the room to Sister's desk. As I walked back to my desk, which was right behind the scrapper's, he stuck his leg out in the aisle to trip me. I saw it before I would have tripped, and stopped. I didn't make a sound, but I looked right at his face and slapped it!

Most of the kids saw and heard the slap, and his response was an audible four-letter expletive. With most eyes and mouths wide open, they looked right up at Sister to see what she would do. I will always remember her reaction. She looked at both of us, not saying a word. I saw her serious eyes and felt them penetrating right through me and my fellow classmate. Not saying a word to us, she smiled, picked up a book and just started reading it. My heart was still pounding hard and fast, but I finished walking to my desk. I had noticed that my classmate turned bright red, but he knew he couldn't do a thing to me. He never tried that again.

Yes, I learned to stick up for myself, and I kept right on facing life's challenges with Dr. Ponseti's words playing in my head, "You will get along just fine Dianne." And I did. Later, I met up with the scrapper at our fifteen-year high school reunion. He reminded me of that moment in seventh grade. Then he apologized for being such a jerk, and we laughed. He also told me that I am the only woman in his life that hit him without him hitting them back—even harder!

MUSIC CONTINUED to be the driving creative energy in me. I always knew I could be a solo singer, but I kept it to myself. I never even told my piano teacher, who taught voice as well as piano. I just sang in the school choir. By seventh grade, I wanted to learn how to play the guitar so I could accompany myself singing.

Folk music was really popular in the 1960's, and I knew many of the folksongs from hearing them on the radio. My dad ordered my first guitar out of a catalog and gave it to me for my thirteenth birthday. It was a junior size, which fit my tiny frame perfectly.

My arms were a challenge as expected, but I taught myself how to strum by using my right thumb to support my right arm, and strumming with my four fingers. I could never use a pic for strumming since my thumb had to support my arm. I managed the left-hand chording just fine with my left arm. I could never play standing up, even with a strap, but I was okay sitting down on a stool or a chair.

Naturally impatient to learn, I was not able to play the guitar right away. With any musical instrument, one has to practice and learn it over time, but I wanted it instantly, so I gave it up until I was going into ninth grade. Then my playing took off, playing and singing as much as time would allow.

In 1968, I went to a movie at the local cinema. The movie had a very popular singer in it. After seeing it, I instantly set my dreams on singing like her! I was sure I could be on the stage some day! One of my favorite songs from that movie spoke right to me. The story was about a young singer who nobody believed could sing, but she could. Everyone told her not to even try because she would never make it. I really identified with the storyline. I learned every one of the movie's songs, because they gave me hope that I could sing on stage someday. I knew people who didn't believe I had talent, much like the movie's main character. And like her, being told she couldn't sing, I believed I could. Whenever anyone told me I couldn't do something or shouldn't try something, it was usually just the push I needed to do it. That naive attitude served me well most of the time, but at other times, I learned the hard way. I learned to listen to reason.

I was a good student, but I had to work very hard to keep my B average. I would get an occasional A, but also an occasional C. I balanced my study time with my piano practice time and lessons.

Music was still my passion, but I also had a flare for the dramatics. My seventh and eighth-grade teacher knew that. She introduced me to the Iowa State Speech Association, and she arranged the very first speech contests for St. Joe's. For the judges, she invited three local high school English teachers. I chose a dramatic reading from the Iowa State Speech Association list, and my teacher entered me into the contests both years. Each year I memorized my pieces, recited them for the judges, and performed to the best of my ability. I was unanimously awarded the highest score allotted by state guidelines both years, and I was definitely hooked on public speaking from that day on. Once I entered high school, those same judges became my English teachers, and they put me on the high school debate and speech team. I continued speaking throughout my high school years, and I attended regional and state contests each year.

As I was getting ready to enter high school, I clearly had a teenager's mindset: high school would be the place to pursue my dreams of singing and performing. Whenever I dreamt of performing, I would forget about my disability. I would get lost in the songs I sang and played on my guitar. I still played the piano, but I never felt secure enough to accompany myself singing. I planned on trying out for the high school choir.

I had many performance goals to achieve in high school, but then something hit me. I was leaving the school I knew every inch of. I was leaving my safety net of wonderful teachers who always accommodated me. I was leaving my small classroom environment for what appeared to me to be a huge building that I had never been in. I had to admit that I was scared, but off I went to my next challenge, attending the public high school in town.

Transferring from class to class was really frightening to me. I didn't think I could do it. The building was three times the size of my parochial school, and it had two stories, just like St. Joe's building did. Once again, my stair-stepping skills would be pushed to their limits. The high school principal arranged a meeting over the summer with my parents and me. It was before the school year began, and he wanted to discuss any problems that my disability might present. The principal was a parishioner at St. Joseph's church and saw me each week at Mass. By observing how I walked, sat and got up from sitting, he knew that maneuvering in and out of high school classes would be hard. So, he made a list of possible solutions and wanted to discuss my options with my parents and me.

We all came up with a good plan for me to get around the building safely. The principal told my teachers what we agreed upon. The plan was for me to leave the classroom five minutes ahead of the other students, so I could get to my next class in time. He explained to my teachers that it would take me longer than the other students to walk to and from classes. He made sure they understood how easy it would be for me to fall if someone ever bumped me during the class transfers. He wanted to avoid that, and so did I. Those extra five minutes were a big safety factor, and I was so thankful I didn't have to fight the crowds. The high school had many more students than St. Joe's ever did. My comfortable small-class environment went from having twelve kids in a class, to having nearly a hundred.

My high school was about the same distance from our house as St. Joseph's was. It was about three blocks away, but not downhill. However, that short walk was still too much for my body to do. My parents, mostly my mom, would drive me every morning and pick me up every afternoon. When she couldn't pick me up, my dad would send one of his employees to come and pick me up. I marvel when I think back at the sacrifices my family made, and all the accommodations the schools made, to make my life so successful. The world didn't have the laws that guided accessibility issues in schools or public places, and yet compassion and common sense provided the accessibility of my world.

I learned early that conserving my energy prevented falls and fatigue. I could do so much more because of that. However, as a child, as well as a teenager, I didn't always agree with or like the limitations my parents put on me. I was quite the typical polio survivor, Type-A personality, and I pushed my limits whenever I could. The Irish spunkiness that I inherited from both my parents, but a little more from my mom's side I think, also served me well in my life's endeavors.

My high school years did offer me many opportunities to perform in the theater department's plays, and I was a part of the choir all four years. I partnered up with one of my friends, and we both played our guitars and sang in harmony for many school and community events. Our big "debut" was when I was in tenth grade and my friend was in ninth. We practiced with our guitars many hours and we came up with great vocal harmony to a popular song, which we performed for the school talent show. Whenever I hear that song, it takes me back to high school. I smile from ear to ear and always sing along with it. We were the girl duo who played at community theater stage breaks, county contests, the country club, as well as family parties.

Performing at family parties had its own issues. As the host of the McTaggart family parties, my father was always announcing, "Dianne will sing everyone a song now," and he would never tell me ahead of time. My Irish temper didn't like that, so there were a couple of times I got even with Dad. The first time was when some neighbors had stopped in to say hi and just wanted to talk to Mom and Dad. They were all sitting in the living room and having a good conversation. I was heading to another room to watch some TV, but I had to walk through the living room in order to get to where the TV was.

I was just as quiet as I could be, but much to my surprise, my dad pulled out my guitar and announced I would sing a song for them. I smiled at Dad, not speaking to him, and sat down with my guitar.

I started to sing a song that had just popped into my head. There had recently been an attempted suicide by someone in town that week, and I had overheard them talking about it when I walked through the room. So I started singing a theme song to a television show about a medical unit in the middle of a war. The theme song lyric mentioned suicide, and it was a perfect song to get even with Dad and show him that the next time he wanted me to sing, he had better let me know ahead of time or I'd embarrass him. When I got to the chorus of the song, the neighbors laughed, but Dad didn't. I took it that I had been successful in making my point to my father. What a brat I could be!

The second time my dad surprised me was at a large family party. There were many friends, store employees, good store customers, as well as my mother's cousin, Bishop Dunn, attending. Mom's cousin was the new bishop for the Catholic Diocese that our parish, St. Joseph's, belonged to. The party had been planned for a long time, and since I was going to the party, I had asked my dad to please not ask me to sing for the group. I explained that I just wanted to enjoy myself like everyone else. He said he understood and would not ask me to sing.

Before the dinner was announced, my dad sprung his surprise announcement, "Listen up everyone, Dianne is going to sing a song before we sit down to eat." Dad had hidden my guitar behind a door, and before I knew it, he had pulled a chair up in the center of the room and handed me my guitar. I gave him quite a look, and Dad just smiled and walked to the far end of the room. So...I thought about what I would sing, and it came to me right away.

I began by tuning my guitar, and said, "Well hello everyone. Are you enjoying yourselves tonight?" They all smiled and nodded, and asked me what was I going to sing? I replied, "Well, this is a song I love to sing. Now the lyrics tell a story, as many songs do, but try to remember while I'm singing that it doesn't really apply to me, but I do love belting out a good sassy song every now and then. Right Dad?" He laughed and nodded his head yes.

I then started to sing a song that told about a young woman who was no longer a virgin!

The whole room, including Bishop Dunn, broke out into laughter. My dad didn't. I really belted the song out good that night, too, but my dad didn't talk to me for at least a week afterward. My mom thought it was funny, probably because she knew I was still a virgin, but she told me I had to apologize to my father, which of course I did.

Looking back on those Dad surprises, I have to admit I never considered my dad's motivation for having me sing for people. It was because he was so proud of me, and of course I knew that, but there was another reason he loved showing me off. Dad once told me that I showed people that I could do some things much better than they ever could. Since he had spent so many hours worrying about me during all those trips to and from the teaching hospital, he had every right to feel the pride of a father. Having me sing was something that made him feel so thankful for getting through all the tough times.

My dad also loved music and was a super singer himself. I know for sure that I inherited my singing talent from him. Dad's voice was very smooth and a blend of some of the most popular male voices on the radio. However, he never sang publicly, just for us family. I once asked him why he didn't join the local barbershop group, since he was certainly good enough. He admitted he was embarrassed because he couldn't read music. I never could convince him that many men, and probably most of the men in that ensemble, couldn't read a note of music. To me and the rest of my family, he was the best singer in the world, and that's what really mattered.

∼

THE SURGERY I had at 12 did help lessen the two-and-a-half-inch difference between my left and right legs. By the end of my tenth-grade year, my right leg's growth had slowed down enough to give my left leg time to catch up a little bit, by one inch. That made my gait easier, and my falls lessened, too. However, all the while I pushed myself to keep up with my peers (and yes, I even surpassed some of them by doing so), my fatigue level was so high at times that occasional falls were inevitable.

As I explained earlier in my story, I could get myself up from falls when I was much younger, but once I grew over four feet tall, I couldn't manage getting up on my own. I had to rely on whoever was around at the time of the fall or wait until someone came along and saw me on the ground. That was hard as a developing teenager. My normal response to falling in those years was embarrassment, mixed with anger at myself.

Adult polio survivors know that life was the sport that caused their joints to wear out. When the polio virus struck the brainstem, which is the center for all the messaging neurons, joints could not be muscularly supported. Joints wear out at a much higher rate when they aren't supported by strong muscle.

Like all other polio survivors who adapted their lives in order to live a normal life, I also adapted. I developed ways of reaching for things that were above my head by using one arm to support the other. I learned how to go up and down stairs with only my right "good" leg to throw my body forward when getting up from low seats, and to use my right arm to pull up and balance my body as I went into a standing position. My right leg always bore the majority of my weight while I stood. I always stood in my choir concerts like everyone else did, but at the end of any concert, my right foot was numb and my leg was throbbing.

Polio survivors were always told we could do it our way and still be contributing to life. We just didn't know the physical price we would pay as the years went on. I never even thought of that. It was all normal for me, and I always thought of myself as able to do anything.

My high school teachers were, for the most part, quite supportive. However, I did run into my first experience of a teacher seeing me as a non-able person while learning how to drive a car. I took the driving class in the summer between ninth and tenth grade.

The school had gotten a car with automatic dimmer switch relays. That meant the driver didn't have to use their left foot to hit the switch on the upper left side of the driver's floor, where the majority of dimmer switches were installed. That was perfect for me, since my left leg was the weaker of the two. The car also had power steering and automatic transmission, so I had no issues with my arms' steering ease and no left clutch issues. My right leg was very able to work the gas and brake pedals.

All summer I learned to drive like the other kids in the class. The teacher never said anything to discourage me, so I was sure I'd pass, which I did. I practiced driving with my parents taking turns teaching me the ropes, and our family friend Steny, who built so many adaptions for me growing up, came up with a hand switch for the left dimmer switch on my parent's car. I had such a positive environment growing up, and as I have aged, I take to adaptions like they are most normal thing in the world.

When my September *sweet sixteenth* birthday rolled around, I was ready to take the driving test to get my driver's license. I had to get a permission slip from my teacher to be able to go down to where the Highway Patrol officer was every Tuesday. The county had to rotate the officer from one small town to another every week, so Tuesday was his day in Elkader.

When I went into class to ask for my permission slip, my teacher looked down and told me not to get my hopes up, because I might not ever be able to drive. I believe my teacher wanted to prepare me for such a possibility. I wanted to scream and cry right then and there, but I just reached out my hand and took the permission slip. As I turned to leave, I said "I believe I can drive, and I'll prove it to you." I then walked out of the classroom and into the empty hallway, which I was ever so happy it was empty, because I broke into tears as I walked.

I headed right outside to my mom's car, where she was waiting to take me for my driving test. Through my tears, I told her what my teacher had just said to me. My mother's determination came right out of her mouth, as she handed me a tissue. She said, "Well I guess you'll show him!"

And I did. Although I was scared to death as I sat in the car with the testing patrol officer in the passenger seat, he was a very calm and quiet man. I explained my disability, and how I needed power steering and automatic transmission for my body to drive barrier free. I demonstrated the dimmer switch challenge with my left leg, but I showed him how I would always position my left leg close enough to the switch in order to work the light dimming when needed.

The officer watched and listened, and we went for the test drive. When we got back to the testing site building, I turned the car off. The officer looked at me kindly, and then he looked down at his clip board. He then asked me to demonstrate again how my left leg could hit the dimmer switch. When I first got into the driver's seat, I had positioned my left leg close enough to the floor switch in order to easily turn the dimmers on and off. I successfully demonstrated my ability to use a normal dimmer switch for the officer.

Once he was finished with the test, he said to me with a big smile, "I don't see any problem with you driving, as long as I put down that power steering and automatic transmission are necessary restrictions. As far as the dimmer switch is concerned, you've got it figured out and need no restriction for that. In my professional judgement, I believe you will be an excellent and safe driver. Congratulations, Dianne."

Oh how I wanted to hug that man, but instead, Mom and I hugged when I came out with my driver's license in hand. I drove myself back to school. Classes were all in session, but I made my first stop at my driving teacher's room. I walked into the room, interrupting the class. I went right up to the teacher, and in front of everyone, I held up my driver's license and said, "I told you I'd do it and I did, so you better watch out when you're crossing the streets now." I immediately turned around and walked out.

As an adult and a retired public school teacher myself, I now shake my head and think of how my teacher could have written me up but didn't. My temper has always been a wild horse I sometimes find hard to tame!

～

As my high school years passed, I took the classes that were in the college-bound track of subjects. My parents always told me I would need a college degree to make a living, since I did not have the ability to work retail or any jobs that would tax my physical capabilities. I knew choosing a college in Iowa was going to be hard, since Iowa winters were not the best place for me to be independent. How would I transfer classes on a large campus with snow and ice? Fortunately, there was one college, and only one, that had a tunnel system between buildings. It was only one hour away from home. Students didn't need to go outside from one end of the campus to the other. The campus was a Catholic all-women's college known as Clarke College (now co-ed Clarke University). With only 400 to 500 women students, it was known for academic excellence and had a terrific music department. Any student applying there had to be both academically qualified and musically gifted in order to audition for acceptance into the music department.

I knew I had the musical gift, but with a strong B average my GPA was still only 3.6. I believed I could apply and try to get in anyway. Many of my teachers encouraged me to do just that. My English teacher and speech coach told me she knew I had the academic quality Clarke required. She offered to write a letter of recommendation for me. My choir director told me that he knew my audition would be flawless and told me not to worry, just sing. However, I soon found out that the school guidance counselor didn't believe like my teachers did.

When junior year college application time rolled around, I

filled out my one choice and hoped for the best, but I needed the school counselor's signature on my transcripts for the application. He requested a meeting with me so we could discuss it. None of my college-bound friends needed a meeting with the guidance counselor for their application process, but I thought he might want to ask me if I had considered the physical demands of college campus life or just talk about my choice and give me some counsel on college life.

When I attended the meeting, he told me not to get my hopes up for acceptance by Clarke College. In reviewing my transcripts, he was of the opinion that my GPA was not high enough for consideration. He counseled me to attend a trade school to get a secretarial position. He believed that would be the most logical way for me to make a living wage with my disability, since I would be able to sit the majority of the time. He knew other students who had attended Clarke College, and it was very academically demanding for many of them. He said they all had been strong A students. I was an occasional A student. He said he would sign my application, but he did not want me to have my hopes up for a good outcome.

Once again, I was told I wasn't able enough. I left with the need to cry, but I was too angry to do it in front of him. I was also too hurt to spout off in my spunky, Irish-temper way. I went into the nearest restroom and had a good cry, and then I left, drying my tears. My temper fueled my resolve to at least try to get into Clarke College.

As I mentioned earlier, I had participated in the Iowa State Speech Association contests from seventh grade through high school. I had a wonderful speech coach, who was also one of my English Literature teachers. She was a very talented orator herself, and she taught her speech students the command of the stage and the power of the English language. She was one of the most influential mentors I have ever had and one of the many teachers that encouraged me to always strive for excellence. She taught me I could do what others thought I couldn't.

I confided in my speech coach about my meeting with the guidance counselor and how it made me feel. She listened to all I had to say and smiled gently saying, "Dianne, you know you can get accepted at Clarke. Your grades are more than average, and your talents are many. So, ignore his advice and apply." She was another person telling me "I could," and I heard my mother's voice say, "Well, I guess you'll show him!"

∽

I DID SHOW HIM. I was accepted to Clarke College into their music department as a full-time music education major. All I really wanted to do was sing and major in vocal performance, but my college advisor explained that a music teaching certificate would come in handy when the "music gigs" were not enough to pay the rent and food bills. Surprisingly, I found the education classes very interesting, and I enjoyed being in the classroom practicums, but I felt something missing in classroom situations for me. I had read about a relatively new area of music study called music therapy. Clarke didn't offer it as a major, but the University of Kansas did offer it as a major, along with Florida State University and Loyola University. I used their college class catalogs to guide me in choosing extra psychology and anatomy classes that a music therapy degree required. I didn't know if I would ever have the opportunity to become a music therapist, but at least I would have some pre-requisite classes done in case I ever did.

My schedule was a demanding one, academically as well as physically, but I pushed forward to achieve my degree. I was smart in choosing Clarke for the physical campus layout. Eastern Iowa winters are long, snowy and full of ice, so having a campus with connected buildings throughout the campus lessened the threat of falling.

On the other hand, there were lots of steps and no elevators and the size of the campus was large for me to walk, so I tired easily. That meant I could and did fall at times. I learned very early on in my life that asking people, most of them complete strangers, to pick me up was a necessity since I seldom fell in a spot where I could pull myself up. I always considered myself a professional "stunt" woman when it came to falling, so I was already experienced in training the lucky devil that came around to pick me up.

At Clarke I was a member of the Clarke-Loras Singers, which was the main Clarke choir. Loras College was started as an all-male college just minutes from the Clarke campus. The two colleges had always had an arrangement to have the men attend music courses at Clarke. Loras had just turned co-ed in the fall of 1971, which was a year before I attended, so Clarke, being an all-female college, needed the men to still attend Clarke choir. Without their attendance, the choir would only be a soprano-alto (SA)-voiced choir. Fortunately, during my entire four years that I sang in the Clarke-Loras Singers, there were enough men to make a vocally balanced mixed choir. I was blessed with the choir director as my main vocal professor and vocal coach, and I earned soloist positions for several of our concerts. He was known as the most demanding vocal instructor, and I learned that his reputation stood true.

I often thought that "demanding" didn't quite describe my college instructor's vocal techniques. Maybe intimidating or scary was more accurate. However, I learned to respect and honor him and his teaching methods and training, which were top-notch!

My vocal abilities grew, and I learned that singing required quite a bit of physical strength. Due to the severity of my spinal curve, I could never stand perfectly straight. I didn't have strong enough muscles. Correct posture is not only extremely difficult for anyone with severe scoliosis, but it's actually impossible. Standing while singing sometimes for hours at a time made me push my muscle strength to its limits.

My passion for singing was the true source of my energy and desire to achieve. I never seemed to care about how my body was hurting. I guess music only fueled that over-achieving trait in me even more. Like one of my favorite historical characters said— *We Can Do It!*

During my freshman and my senior years of study, I had several opportunities to travel and go on spring break choir tours. The first tour was to the East Coast, which included singing on the U.S. Capitol steps in Washington, D.C. as well as singing in Harlem in New York City and some venues in Philadelphia. Of course, those bus tours had unique physical tests for me. Bus steps were REALLY hard to make, but I adapted my way on and off the bus. I would kick my right leg (good leg) up onto the step and grab ahold of the railing with both arms. I'd then pull my body up with all my might and get my weaker, left leg up next. I would do that for every step until I was safely inside the bus. I always waited for everyone to be on the bus before me so I didn't have to worry about holding up someone from entering the bus. By the end of all of my bus tours, I had the bus drivers reaching out to lend me a hand. They watched, sometimes in awe, when I first entered their bus. They figured out that if I reached for their hand, it was easier on my arms than using the railing. Today I realize while looking back that I have been given so many instances of helpful people all along the way, and boy, do I feel blessed.

Some days we would have more than one concert performance, so my legs were throbbing and weak after those concerts. I was always determined to do everything everyone else did. I remember several times when my legs would give out as we would be walking to and from venues or sightseeing, and I would fall to the ground. However, I trained all the men in the choir to pick me up safely with a "Dianne technique" I had perfected throughout my lifetime.

I would train anyone that offered to pick me up to always put their arms directly under my arms to hoist me up and wait for me to count to three. That allowed me time to position myself to get my legs in a good position for standing. If anyone tried to pick me up with their arms circled around my waist, much lower than I needed, it would hurt my back. Once standing, I just brushed myself off, caught my breath and kept going. It didn't matter how my body felt, because I was part of the choir and never missed a performance. Type-A personality— but at times, Type-A+ personality.

The New York City leg of my first tour was quite eventful for me, and it was the first time this little Iowa girl was exposed to a huge city like the Big Apple. We checked into a hotel in the heart of Broadway, since we had two nights to see a real Broadway play in between our scheduled choir concerts. As soon as we had unloaded the bus, we all headed to Radio City Music Hall to see the famous dancers.

Radio City Music Hall was about four blocks from our hotel. City blocks were like miles to me. I was already exhausted from the Washington, D.C. part of the tour, but I didn't want to miss anything. I was probably twenty feet away from our hotel walking with the group, when a panhandler came up to me hitting my arm, and said, "Hey, help out a fellow cripple, would ya?" I was instantly in shock and didn't know how to respond to him. All of a sudden, two of the male tenors came up behind me, and each took one of my arms and hailed a cab. They told me to get in and asked the cabby to take us to Radio City Music Hall. Well, this was a New York cabby after all, and he thought we were crazy because it was so close and not worth his time. My two tenor friends replied in a very New York-way, and that cab ride was the fastest ride I ever had.

Not only did I get to see Radio City Music Hall, but I saw my first Broadway plays. One of the plays had a very popular actress I grew up watching in the movies. I was so tickled to have the chance to see stars like her. All my teenage fantasies of singing on the stage came flooding back to me. I felt like I was in my own dream.

One final note of my 1973 New York spring break tour: I have always had to look down as I walk to avoid possible falls—I still do. The smallest dent in a walkway or an obstacle like twigs or pebbles, can throw my balance off, and down I go. Since New York City was and still is a very fast-paced city, I had never been in an environment like this before. It was a huge threatening obstacle course in which I realized I could be knocked down in a flash everywhere I walked. Coming back to my hotel from the theater after seeing a matinee, I was walking as carefully as possible, when a man swerved on the sidewalk just in time to catch me from falling right into him. I looked up as he said in a wonderful British accent, "Are you ok dear?" I embarrassingly replied, "Yes, thank you." I recognized him immediately. I was a big fan of a television series about British spy agents, and I faithfully watched it for years. It was *Patrick MacNee*, the lead actor in that series who prevented my fall and caught me! I have told that story to many of my family and friends as my real-life experience with a British knight in shining armor. It was another huge thrill for this small-town gal from Iowa!

The Midwest choir trip to the East Coast turned out to be a wonderful experience for me. Though it was a physically draining trip, there were lots of fond memories and personal growth as a person, as well as a musician.

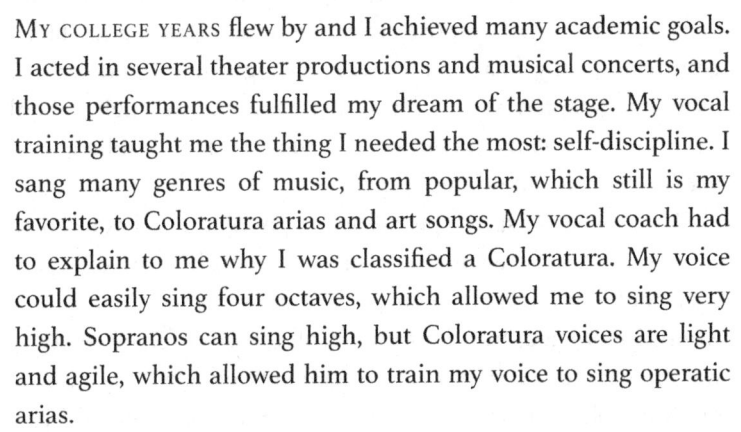

My college years flew by and I achieved many academic goals. I acted in several theater productions and musical concerts, and those performances fulfilled my dream of the stage. My vocal training taught me the thing I needed the most: self-discipline. I sang many genres of music, from popular, which still is my favorite, to Coloratura arias and art songs. My vocal coach had to explain to me why I was classified a Coloratura. My voice could easily sing four octaves, which allowed me to sing very high. Sopranos can sing high, but Coloratura voices are light and agile, which allowed him to train my voice to sing operatic arias.

One of my biggest challenges, vocally and physically, was being the high soprano soloist for Handel's Messiah concert in my senior year at Clarke. Since I really loved singing in coffee houses and bars, my vocal coach had a huge job, much like breaking a wild horse, convincing me that I could sing as a Coloratura. I did it much to my own surprise, and I loved the rigors classical training demanded. When I wasn't practicing to sing as a Coloratura, I performed in small venues with my guitar and occasionally with a piano accompanist which allowed me to sing one of my favorite musical styles, the blues.

The Messiah concert was hours long, and I stood for the entire concert. I remember how my legs and feet were numb afterward. It is amazing to me now that I never asked to sit down. I truly believed I could be like everyone else, so it never occurred to me at the time. That was the level of denial I had, and it continued to be a strong coping mechanism throughout most of my life.

I completed my B.A. in Music Education, as well as my student teaching requirements. I taught for six weeks in an elementary school, and six weeks in a middle and high school.

Since my arms could not conduct as every music student is trained to conduct, using sweeping arm movements to direct, I developed my own, adaptive style of conducting using my facial gestures and my head, along with my right hand and wrist. I used my adapted style of conducting with the high school choirs, but I really hated it. I needed to feel fulfilled, and teaching music did not fulfill me.

I wanted to inspire special-needs populations. I wanted to show them that even if they weren't made like everyone else, they could still achieve their goals. I knew music therapy was where I belonged, but the thought of going on for more study was almost too much for me. I resigned myself to getting a music teaching job somewhere in Iowa, as soon as I graduated. I had the application for an Iowa Teacher's Certificate ready to complete once I had my B.A. in hand.

Although my vocal coach encouraged me to apply for graduate school, I didn't. I knew my parents had paid enough tuition after four years of a private, non-state institution. That was enough money spent for me, and I was ever so grateful to them. They made such a sacrifice for me to get my college education. I had always known that level of love and support from them my whole life. However, God had a divine plan for me, or I like to call it a *divine blueprint*, made out long in advance.

My last choir tour would be a fateful turning point in my career. After graduation day, May 8, 1976, the Clarke-Loras Singers were scheduled to tour Poland for three weeks as U.S. youth representatives. An international youth organization had a request from the Socialistic Students Union in Poland to have three different U.S. college music ensembles be their guests for a three-week tour. We were also invited to study at the Music Conservatory in Krakow, Poland, as well as perform in Warsaw and in Lublin, Poland. The Clarke-Loras Singers were chosen, along with an all-male college choir from Arkansas, and a youth orchestra from Winter Haven, Florida.

Since we were all from different areas of the United States, we traveled on our own separate route first. We all joined up in a single group at JFK Airport in New York City. All together we were the international youth representatives, representing the United States of America. From there, we boarded our chartered jet together.

As I mentioned earlier, this tour was in 1976, and it was our unfortunate luck to be flying when the nation's Federal Air Traffic Controllers' strike was on. We were supposed to fly direct to Warsaw from New York, but got re-routed and landed in the Copenhagen, Denmark. We were told that we would be there for at least twelve to twenty-four hours until the flight could be routed safely to Poland.

As the true college kids that we were, we just hunkered down and slept on the floor, and checked out the cafes and bars in the Danish airport. We decided to see if Danish beer was as good as our favorite American ones were. Getting prematurely grounded gave us a great opportunity to mingle with the other groups and get to know them all. I had only flown round-trip one time before this, from Chicago to Detroit on a small airplane that flew out of Midway, the smaller of the two Chicago airports. This European tour was quite the adventure for me. We were finally routed to Warsaw after about a fifteen-hour delay. Off we flew, and we landed just fine in Warsaw.

Visiting Poland was such an incredible opportunity. It was still a communist country, and we saw military guards with rifles at the airport when we landed. We had all been given an orientation before leaving New York, that explained we should expect armed guards visible at many places for all three weeks of the tour. Our Polish hosts, the Socialistic Students' Union, sent members to the airport to welcome us as we arrived. They were just like any college-age students, excited to meet us and were very welcoming.

We were told that a chartered bus would take us all around the country for our performances, as well as for our sightseeing times. Our director told us to remember that all of our buses, as well as our hotel rooms and classrooms at the conservatory, would more than likely be bugged with surveillance equipment. I knew I would have to keep my big mouth in check.

Our choir director threatened to tell our parents, and anyone else he could, if we "misbehaved." We needed to maintain the proper U.S. diplomatic behaviors at all times. Okay, college-age perfect angels—probably not, but I knew that the soldiers I saw had loaded rifles and were everywhere we went, so that helped keep us in line...most of the time.

We knew we could not drink any water from the taps, unless we wanted to stay on the commode for three weeks, so we learned to make do. I learned two of the most convenient Polish words, Dziękuję, which means thank you, and Piwo, which means beer! I was also very happy that I followed the travel packing tips we were given—pack your own toilet paper—because, wow, theirs was cardboard. And we were told to pack prescription-strength Lomotil, which is a very good human radiator seal. Okay, enough about water and commodes. How did I get from Poland to my music therapy degree? I said it was a fateful turning point in my life. That's the story to come.

PART III

MUSIC THERAPY AND BEYOND

3

The Polish choir tour was filled with concerts, sightseeing and days of study at the Music Conservatory in Krakow. I made many new friends from our fellow international youth organizations, especially with the Winter Haven, Florida Youth Orchestra. Our Clarke-Loras Singers socialized with the Winter Haven orchestra. Four members of the orchestra were the children of the director. They became my good friends. All four of them were terrific musicians, in and out of the concerts. Our groups would get together for jam sessions after concerts and days of study. I loved singing jazz and popular music during those fun sessions, with many accompanied by my Winter Haven friends.

Two of them attended Florida State University (FSU) in Tallahassee. I was quite familiar with FSU. Since Clarke didn't offer a music therapy major, I used FSU's catalog listings of music therapy curriculum as my guide when choosing classes at Clarke. I told my Florida friends about my desire to be a music therapist, and why I couldn't get that degree at Clarke. They told me FSU had a super music therapy graduate program, and they kept reminding me throughout our three weeks together. They kept saying I should apply for my Master's degree. I had known of the program for years. It was highly rated in the music therapy world. I had a dream that if I could go to graduate school it would have to be in a warm climate, with no ice and snow. I could be independent only in that climate.

The more my new Florida friends talked about FSU and how they would be there if I needed anything, the more I began to believe I could do it. However, we wouldn't get back to the United States until June 21st. How could I even think of getting my application in on time and be accepted for the fall semester, which would begin the second week of September? Most important of all, how could I ask my parents to pay for two more years of study and be over 1200 miles away? How could I leave my family to go to a different state, where there wouldn't be any family around? It wouldn't be an hour drive to home, like the past four years at Clarke. However, the more I thought about it, the more I believed in my dream. I left Poland more determined than ever to at least try. My Winter Haven friends said, "Dianne, you can do it!" So, I declared full speed ahead!

~

I DISCUSSED my desire to study music therapy with my parents as soon as I arrived home. As always, they supported the idea and told me to try. I sent away for the application to FSU the third week in June. I received it in the mail right after July 4th. Fortunately, I had already taken the GRE, the Graduate Records Examination, in the second semester of my senior year at Clarke. FSU required all graduate applicants to submit their GRE exam score. I had taken the exam just in case an opportunity ever arose in my future.

The memory of my high school guidance counselor telling me I didn't have what it took for college popped into my head, even though I knew I had already proven him wrong. I graduated from college with an above-average grade point, plus I had already received my Iowa Teacher's Certificate. Yet even with those accomplishments, it struck me as funny how those few negative memories clouded my self-confidence.

Fortunately, all the voices of the "somebodies" in my life who said *I could* took over. I sent off my completed application the second week of July. I heard from the FSU Graduate Department School of Music by the end of July. They had accepted me on the contingency that my music audition would be up to their standards. They scheduled my audition for the day after my birthday, September 9th.

Leaving Iowa was a big milestone in my life. Leaving my family was the hardest. As my mother put it, "Out of all the five kids in the family, I never thought you would be the one to move far away." My entire family always protected me. I asked my older brother Pat how it was having me as a sister, and he said, "We hope we made you feel special," which they all did. I knew then, and I know now, that they waited on me all the time, grabbing things, helping me up big steps, and so many more loving acts.

My parents told me that I had to believe in my independence more than ever if I wanted to be a music therapist. I threw away my original plan to apply for teaching positions around the state of Iowa right after the Polish choir tour was over. Once I received my FSU acceptance, I applied for and received a Florida Teacher's Certificate. I thought if I didn't cut it in graduate school, I could always teach music. I knew being a teacher in Florida weather would be much better than teaching in Iowa weather.

During my last semester at Clarke, I completed my student teaching. I had to drive 25 miles to my assigned school. That semester was enough to show me that achieving my independence in Iowa was going to be next to impossible. Driving to and from school on ice and snow could be done, very carefully. However, walking from my car to the school would always be a gamble, with a very high price to pay for my body. Since I was getting older, my falls were not as easy to take. My knees and ankles were already loaded with arthritis. Taking a teaching job would be difficult, but I wanted to show my parents their investment was worth it. I also wanted to prove to myself that "I Can Do It!"

Going to graduate school was a dream come true. I felt bad that I was such a financial burden on my parents. My dad wouldn't listen to anything regarding that. He told me that he and Mom would drive down to Tallahassee with me in my blue Mercury Comet. He and Mom wanted to find an apartment with me, move me in, and get me settled. Once that was accomplished, they would fly home.

Off to Tallahassee we went, and we arrived on my twenty-third birthday, September 8, 1976. There happened to be two Elkader Central Community High School graduates who lived and worked in Tallahassee. My parents knew them both. One was a professor at the FSU School of Law, and another one was an attorney who lived and practiced in Tallahassee. Dad felt better knowing that if I ever got in trouble, I could call those Iowa guys. Our joke was that at least these two guys would.know how to post bail for me!

We looked up the attorney the day we arrived, and he took us out to lunch. Afterwards he showed us apartments that he knew were close to the school. They were directly across the street from the law school. Most graduate students and law students lived at that apartment complex, so it was a more studious environment. That same day we signed a year's lease. I was worried about signing a lease, since my audition wasn't until the next day. However, my parents never doubted my musical talents, and they told me they were sure I was going to be accepted.

They were right. My audition was scary, but I sang two of the more difficult pieces from my senior recital at Clarke during my last semester there. The top FSU vocal coach specifically requested me to be her student. I was so honored. However, when I signed up for my music therapy classes, I could not fit her schedule availability into my class schedule. She tried to talk me into switching to a voice performance principal for my Master's program, but I knew I was meant to be a music therapist. I found another vocal coach who fit into my schedule. I was all set to begin my new life at FSU.

My father left the day after I moved into the apartment, and my mom stayed on to help me unpack and see me through my first full week. I decided to get a roommate to help with the rent. I put up a bulletin board advertisement at the entrance of the University. The girl who responded was moving in the following week. That's when Mom scheduled her plane ride home. She knew there would only be room for two in my small, one bedroom apartment.

When the time came for Mom to leave, I drove her to the airport. We both broke down and cried as we said goodbye. My mom was never known for crying. She was always very strong, and I always followed her lead when facing life's tests, but this time was different. I felt such a flood of mixed emotions. She was feeling them, too. We both knew that from this moment on, I would be living the independent life she and Dad had always wanted for me. The female doctor who told my parents at my birth, the one who advised my parents to put me in a crippled childrens' home, was definitely wrong. It was true that my Iowa home, family, and friends would be miles away, but I was starting out on a great adventure.

Amidst our tears, Mom and I hugged and said goodbye.

Mom told me that she loved me, and to remember she and Dad always believed I could do whatever my mind was set on doing. As she walked away, she turned and said, "Don't forget we are only a phone call away." With tears in my eyes I nodded and said, "I know, Mom."

When I got back to my apartment from the airport, I immediately got busy studying and reviewing my class notes that I had taken during my first week. Classes were more demanding than I was used to, but I loved the demands. I knew I would be more than okay in Tallahassee. I didn't dwell on my mom's goodbye as I studied, but as the time went by and evening began, I decided to call home...I had to check on Mom.

~

Florida was a perfect place for me to become a music therapy student. I lived only two blocks from the School of Music buildings. I still had to drive to classes, but I parked in a special assigned parking space. The year was 1976, and the Americans with Disabilities Act (ADA) was not yet the law at state universities. I knew I had to be my own advocate and ask for what I needed. I went to the Registrar's Office requesting a special parking space, one that would be assigned to me. This was a brand-new world for me, and a much larger one than I had ever experienced.

I was beginning to recognize my limitations, or as I prefer to say, my boundaries. I had to speak up for my special needs. I knew my chances of falling would increase if I walked to and from class each day, but even knowing this, there were a handful of times I fell anyway. On one of the last times I walked to class, I learned a big lesson when I fell. As I had done so often in the past, I waited for a stranger to come along and pick me up. My embarrassment brought me back to my senses. I stuck to my driving/parking privilege and was very grateful for it. I was so happy that I had such a short distance to walk from the parking space to my classes.

I never took accommodations for granted. I felt blessed to be listened to and assisted. During the pre-ADA era, many people with disabilities were ignored. Reflecting back on my childhood and education, I marvel at all the accommodations my parents, teachers, and friends made for my disability. Those accommodations lifted barriers and gave me my love of independence.

I do not make light of the many advocates' hard work who made the ADA a reality. They made incredible advancements in the world of disability, and the ADA changed the world for the better. I have often said to family and friends that if I had to be born with a disability, this is a great time to be alive.

The music therapy curriculum was challenging, but I loved every bit of it. I was assigned practicums, which were much like student teaching, at special schools, hospitals, and rehabilitation facilities. They exposed me to various populations and gave me wonderful music therapy experiences. Those populations included the mentally retarded (now identified as Intellectually Challenged), learning disabled, physically disabled, and the emotionally/mentally challenged. The practicums had a wide range of ages as well, from infants to the elderly.

I worked hard and learned much about the gift of music therapy. As I worked, I realized that my talents were always meant to be used to help others, not just for my own pleasure and entertainment.

In order to complete a Master's degree program, I was required to complete a graduate thesis. My last six months of the two-year program was spent as a full-time music therapy intern at a state mental hospital in Georgia. It was there that I collected data for my thesis.

Mental patients were often housed in special state facilities back in 1978. Many of the patients were involuntarily committed by their families, and many were labeled as schizophrenics. There were only two kinds of wards in the hospital, locked wards and open wards. The most volatile patients were in the locked wards. They were highly medicated, and many had gone through electric shock therapy, which was used on them in the late 1950's and 1960's. I chose my thesis subjects to be the schizophrenic patients from the locked ward. They would not only be my test group, but they'd also be my control group. I gave the test-group clients a list of topics to choose from. From their list, they were told to create poetic words or stories. I then took their ideas and created a song on the guitar while in our group therapy sessions.

The control group would be given the same list of topics and asked to create poetic words or stories. However, I did not put their ideas to music. The non-music control subjects had much less verbal participation or interest compared to the test group who had their ideas made into songs. I wanted to measure the effects of music therapy on the number of verbalizations made by that special population.

I won't bore you with the entire scientifically-designed project and all the data I collected, but I will say that I observed marked positive responses with the majority of the test subjects. Patients who had been non-verbal for many years began to verbalize in a singing style. Some who believed they lived on another planet helped make up lyrics that were very *earthly and realistic*, which I put to music. Socially, the test group began to interact with each other, instead of sitting in their chairs rocking back and forth, staring at the floor. I felt my new occupation was going to be the most exciting thing I could ever imagine.

During my internship, I met and worked with patients that were on the open wards as well. My music therapy supervisor conducted reality therapy sessions with the open-ward patients.

As my supervisor, she had me observe her sessions in the beginning of my internship. I then was assigned to lead the sessions for the last two months of my term. I learned reality therapy group techniques and dynamics, which I loved leading. My supervisor said I was a natural, and the patients opened up to me easier than she had ever observed before.

One of the male patients in the group, whom I will call David, had been hospitalized for nineteen years. He told me his parents put him there when he was seventeen years old. He was a very pleasant man and not volatile or dangerous at all. In my reality therapy sessions, I used music as a mode of therapy for the patients to feel safe enough to open up and share their thoughts. David shared that he loved Elvis songs. He said, "Sometimes I have a radio in my head that plays Elvis's music. I always have to dance to it," which explained why David was almost always in motion. I learned to play several Elvis Presley songs on the guitar for him, and it always made David dance and smile.

Along with therapy sessions, music therapy interns had to manage a token store. The store was set up by the music therapy department, along with the supervisors of all the open wards. Patients earned tokens for their good behavior on the wards, and they used their tokens at the store for treats like candy, soda or tobacco products. The store was nothing but a storage closet with a horizontally divided door inside the music therapy building, which was a free-standing building detached from the main hospital.

One day while I was manning the token store, David came to shop. He was quite talkative and happy that day. He said, "I want to tell you something." When all the other customers had left, he said, "I think I'm Jesus." I immediately asked, "Why do you think you're Jesus, David?" He replied, "Because I read a book about schizophrenia, and it said that many schizophrenics believe they are Jesus. The book calls it a Jesus complex." I nodded and continued to listen. He continued, "Since all of my doctors say I have schizophrenia, I must be Jesus." I then asked him, "David, have you ever done or thought "bad" things?" He nodded and rattled off a number of "bad" things he had done. Now, if I listed all of David's "bad" things here, my story would be labeled—FOR ADULTS ONLY. Just take my word for it—BAD is a nice word for some of what he shared with me that day! However, I knew him to be a very well-behaved patient. There was never a problem written in his entire file. So I asked him, "Does Jesus sin?" He looked me straight in the eye and immediately replied, "No, never." I looked straight at him and said, "Then you can't be Jesus." It was one of the best moments I had during my internship. He said that nobody had ever told him that. He always wondered why he had urges to sin, being Jesus. We had quite a discussion that day.

Throughout my time at the hospital, I worked with a team of medical professionals. It included psychiatrists, therapists, and social workers. I discussed David's case with the team in one of our weekly meetings, and I asked if the team could re-evaluate him. I thought that David could be released from the hospital and placed in a supervised group home. I wasn't sure if it was possible to find such a placement, especially after nineteen years of living in an institution. However, after a month of searching and interviewing prospective group home supervisors, I found one in a city two hours away from the hospital. The home had availability for two males. Since I also worked with another male patient who was very much like David, I had the team evaluate both David and the other male. The team found both patients suitable for group home living and told me to set up their release from the hospital. I used many music therapy sessions to prepare them for living together in a group home. These men were teens when they were committed to the state hospital and were scared to leave. We worked through their fears, and they eventually became excited about a new, full life of possibilities. The day I drove them off the hospital grounds, after nearly twenty years of living there, I watched their faces and knew—music therapy was my chosen field.

I HAD many more experiences as a music therapy intern. Looking back on them now, I'm happy to say they made my life easier to live. The sum of one's experiences do shape life's future decisions. With the attitude my parents instilled in me, believing I could do anything I wanted to do but differently than others, I chose to work with some dangerous patients. It never entered my mind that they might perceive me as more vulnerable than other hospital workers.

One of those patients was a man on the locked ward, who I will call Ron. The psychiatrist in charge of the locked ward asked me to work with him, to try to reach him through music therapy techniques. I was told he had been a violent patient when he was first admitted, but his medications had controlled his outbursts for several years. The psychiatrist felt as long as the medication was working so well, I would be safe working with him. Being young and confident—and a little stupid, I think—I never thought about the possibility of being hurt. I knew male orderlies were always around the locked ward, so I knew I'd be fine. I accepted the challenge and began Ron's music therapy treatment plan.

At our first session, he didn't talk much. Since he was highly medicated, I expected a subdued response. I put relaxing music on in the background, and asked Ron to draw what came into his mind with the music. He drew many violent pictures. One was of a very large man choking a woman with blood all around her. The woman in the picture was very small. I asked who the man and woman were in the picture. He told me he was the man, and the woman was his mother. I calmly ended our therapy session and left the ward. I was very happy the locked ward was always locked. I showed the psychiatrist the pictures and reported details of the session. He gave me Ron's file to read, so that I could come back and discuss it with him. It turns out that Ron's mother was a schizophrenic herself. She admitted him to the hospital over fifteen years ago with the help of the police, after she had been attacked by her son.

When I went back to discuss Ron's file with the psychiatrist, he told me he had prescribed medications months earlier that were working very well. They had reduced the patient's violent outbursts completely. He was hoping music therapy might be a good mode of therapy for Ron. However, after our discussion of Ron's drawings, along with notes I had taken while observing him during our session, the psychiatrist decided to cancel all future sessions. My music therapy supervisor agreed with that decision as well. We all knew that the possible violent behavior was not controlled enough for taking a risk to any music therapist. I totally agreed with their decision!

The time at the mental hospital passed quickly, and I was coming to the end of my six-month internship. Some renovations were being done to the hospital, which required the token store to move temporarily to an old, unused section of the hospital. That section was still physically connected but away from the main, functional part of the hospital. While repairs were being done, the intercom system was temporarily inactive in the unused areas. My supervisor thought that, for the short time we needed the area for the token store, it would still be a safe enough location. So did I. After all, the token store was only open for one hour a day, so I didn't give it much thought when I went for my shift.

Somebody Told Me I Could

It was one of my last days working at the token store, and not many patients came. I assumed they skipped it because it was a longer walk from their wards. I was disappointed. I was hoping to say goodbye to some of my regular patients and wish them well. As I started locking up and turning off the lights, Ron, the locked-ward patient, jumped out of a closet. I didn't scream. Somehow I remained calm. He looked at me silently, occasionally twitching, but didn't move much.

"Oh Ron," I said "I am so glad you're here. My supervisor wants me to put these heavy oak chairs on top of all the tables." Still shaking inside I pointed to my left and said, "I'm so weak. Lifting these chairs is really hard for me, and you're so much stronger than I am. It's a lucky thing you're here. Maybe you could help me with these? You're so strong, I bet it'll be easy for you to lift."

Inside I was shaking all over. As I physically picked up a nearby oak chair making a grunting sound, I could feel my heart racing, but I knew I needed to look helpless. I remembered some tips I had learned while attending a lecture on rape during my junior year at college. I learned that a rapist wants to violently subdue his victim knowing he has all the strength between the two. I thought if I continued to play weak and helpless, I could get away. With no intercom and no nearby staff, I just prayed that my creative wit would be enough.

Ron did pick up a couple of chairs and placed them on the table. All the while I was doing the same, making small talk the whole time. He never spoke a word. All of a sudden, he threw a chair to the floor and ran out of the room like a lightning bolt, heading for the outside hospital grounds.

Since I could not run, let's say I used every fiber in my being to rush to the nearest hospital employee, who happened to be a janitor. I told him what had just happened. He ran and got ahold of a nurse. He told her to go to the intercom system and report the locked-ward patient running loose on the grounds. I immediately sat down in the nearest safe area, and just stared off into space, saying to myself, "What the hell were you thinking, Dianne?" Hours later they found the patient in a truck he had stolen from a nearby Army truck station and brought him back to the hospital heavily sedated. I never dreamt a music therapist could or would ever have such adventures. However, I did. I even had a few more through the years, too!

~

I MET my future husband during the second year of my graduate study. October, 1977. Dennis and I met at a prayer group at the Catholic church we both attended. My girlfriend and I played guitars and sang for the group. Dennis had just moved to Tallahassee after graduating from law school in Gainesville, Florida. His sister suggested he go to one of the new, charismatic prayer groups that were just starting up. She told him it would be a good place to meet nice girls, instead of in bars. She was right. It ended up being a good place for me to meet a nice guy too. We were married in November 1978.

I finished my course work at FSU and defended my thesis in August of 1978. I had to wait for my Master's degree diploma to arrive in the mail, since I had to go to work after securing a job in Orlando, Florida. Orlando, being five hours away from Tallahassee, was too far to drive to my graduation ceremony. I was okay with that, since securing a job in music therapy was quite difficult. There were very few hospitals that recognized music therapy as a treatment modality, and special schools for various disabilities didn't recognize music therapists, just music educators. I was lucky I had applied for and received my Florida Teacher's Certificate when I moved to Florida.

My first job was at a Catholic school for Down Syndrome

and learning-disabled children. The salary was half of what the public schools offered teachers, but there were no openings for a music teacher in the public schools, let alone a music therapist with a graduate degree. It was a very good beginning job for me. They were able to hire me as a teacher, not a music therapist, due to the diocese requirement of hiring only certified teachers. Because I was certified, the principal was happy the school got a music therapist, since they had requested that in the first place.

Dennis secured an associate's job in a law firm in downtown Orlando. The firm had just broken away from another firm. He was the first associate hired, and the sixth attorney on board. He was excited to get in on the ground floor of a new start-up. He had passed the bar in June while working for the Florida Attorney General's Office in Tallahassee. We were both starting our first real jobs. Our years of studying were finally going to be put to good use.

I was lucky to secure a job before we moved to Orlando. During his last year of law school, in 1975, Dennis had a summer clerking position in one of the big Orlando firms. That summer job provided him with a strong network of Orlando business associates he relied on for employment recommendations. Thanks to those contacts, he began work in October 1978. We also chose to live in Orlando because Dennis's parents lived there in a condominium. I was happy to be near family again, even though it was my future family. My life was rooted in the importance of family, so I loved the idea of moving to Orlando. Dennis lived with his parents from the time we arrived in August until our wedding in November. I moved into the apartment we rented. I was soon going to be in my new Wall family.

Our November wedding was in Iowa over Thanksgiving vacation. Just starting new jobs, we didn't have any vacation time. A blizzard hit on Thanksgiving Day, the day before our wedding. We were lucky that the wedding was on a Friday night, because the county snowplows cleared the roads enough for most guests and relatives to attend safely.

Most couples remember their wedding nights for obvious reasons. However, we remember ours for completely different reasons. After the wedding reception, we drove to the nearest small city that had motels, and arrived around 11:30 p.m. that night. When we got to the place, it was only twenty degrees outside, and the entire place, including our "honeymoon suite," — had NO HEAT. We slept in layers of pants and sweaters and our winter coats! Needless to say, we checked out at 7:00 a.m. the next morning and drove about four miles down the highway to another motel that was fully heated. We love laughing and telling our honeymoon story now, but not then. We only had a warm motel room for one night of our two-night honeymoon, but it became another laughable memory.

When we checked in at the warmer motel, the front desk manager said, "Wow, think of this. The people next door to you have the same last name as yours." We looked at each other and laughed. Dennis asked, "Did that Wall family have a baby with them?" The manager replied, "Yes, they did." At that point, Dennis and I knew it was Peter, his brother and best man at our wedding, and his wife and baby girl. When we got to our room, we knocked on their door yelling, "Hey you guys, there's going to be a pizza party next door while the Notre Dame Fighting Irish play the University of Southern California Trojans on TV." Peter came to the door laughing and said, "Well, this is a helluva honeymoon, but I know you guys would never miss Dennis's alma mater, ND!" We all ordered out for pizza that afternoon and celebrated our honeymoon—*family-style*! I always laugh when I look back on that memory. It's not every couple that can say their honeymoon was a family affair.

We all checked out that Sunday morning together. My brother Kevin was waiting outside the motel. He had made the hour's drive from Elkader so he could drive us to the airport to catch our flights home. Dennis and I were going back to work the next day in Orlando—to seventy-degree weather. Peter and his family were going back to upstate New York—twenty degrees and snow. As Dennis and I were boarding our plane, we smiled at each other knowing that we would miss my Iowa family, but we would NEVER miss blizzards.

∼

I STAYED at my first school job for only one year. I had developed asthma and was quite sick with respiratory issues, so I knew I needed to get stronger. We found a condominium to rent a few months after the school year ended.

My asthma cleared up right after we moved. It turned out that our first apartment was next to an orange grove, and that was the allergen that triggered my asthma. I also had two orange trees in the courtyard right outside my first classroom!

Looking back, I know I would have moved on to another job after only one year anyway, because the principal didn't truly understand music therapy. I was only used as a music teacher. I loved the students, but knew I was needed in another place. After leaving my first job, I healed quite well and got stronger in a short time.

I then took a job with the public school system in Orlando, as a music therapist for their Adult Education program. It was only part-time, but there were no other music therapy positions available. The job required driving to special schools for adult mentally-challenged adults, as well as Senior Centers that offered music lessons and choirs for their elderly. I loved all my music therapy clients, in every different setting. I had to haul many musical instruments around in the trunk of my car. It was physically challenging, but I found creative ways to get the instruments inside the buildings. For example, the senior housing project I went to each week for sing-alongs and music lessons had a grocery cart the residents used to get their groceries up to their apartments. Each week the manager of the building made sure the cart was available for me to unload my car of instruments. At another one of my sites, the director always had a hand cart waiting for me to use. Wherever my assignments took me, people were always willing to help.

After working for over a year in the Adult Education Department of the county public school system, my name was given to the director of the elementary/secondary music department. There was a sudden vacancy for a substitute music therapist-music teacher at a special school designed for emotionally and mentally-challenged students, along with learning disabled. This school was first grade through middle school. It was created for the placement of students who could not learn in their regular, neighborhood schools. The year was 1980, and "mainstreaming" (better known as inclusion now) was not the educational model. Educators then believed that children with various disabilities needed to be in their own specialized schools. Those schools, such as the one I was considering, had special education teachers and therapists who were specialized and dedicated to the needs of specific populations. This school was designed for three different populations. One group of students was labeled Severely Emotionally Disturbed, or SED, and the second group was labeled Learning Disabled, or LD. The third group was composed of autistic students.

Their full-time music teacher had a sudden illness, requiring her to take leave from October through December and possibly longer. I decided that it was an opportunity to get my foot in the door for a future full-time teaching or therapy position in the public schools. The traveling required in my part-time adult education job was getting very physically draining, so although this was only a three-month substitute position, I believed I should do it.

When I met the school principal, he told me that I had to put on a Christmas show for the Parent-Teacher Association (PTA) in the second week of December. I told him I could do it. The regular music teacher warned me that she had not started anything for Christmas yet. She told me most students could not read above a second or third-grade level, which made reading lyrics very difficult. Also, no student could read music. As usual, that didn't faze me. I started the job the second week in October, and even with the "testing" of their new substitute by every child in the school, we had a great Christmas program.

That challenge wasn't quite the typical substitute teacher experience. As I previously mentioned, the school population had SED students. The principal and assistant principal were often summoned by classroom teachers to come and retrieve students who acted out in class. All classrooms had an intercom in the room. Some of the examples of acting out were unique to that particular school, such as a student would decide to hold a scissors to the throat of a fellow classmate, or a student would leave the classroom and go up on the school building's roof for some fresh air. The principal once told me if he ever left his job as principal, he could be a professional roofer since he was so good at climbing up after the students. All teachers had to have excellent disciplinary skills in order to work at that special school. Teachers and therapists could never maintain a decent learning environment without them.

As the music therapist, I had every student in the school for their music class once or twice a week. My classroom was a portable classroom away from the main school, so I was happy that the intercom worked well. It was a portable building detached from the school, and there were three steps to make to get in or out of it. I found I could manage the steps since it had a sturdy railing.

As a substitute teacher for a few months, I didn't think I could ask for an accessible accommodation. I remember when the principal took me to the music building on my interview, he asked if the steps would be something I could do. I reassured him I could. I was very grateful for that railing, because I used my arms to balance and pull myself up. Being only 27 years old, PPS had not yet manifested in me, so I knew I could do the steps.

The kids used many techniques to test me, from throwing chairs at me to hurling verbal, obscene threats—some quite colorful. A few kids threw tantrums on the floor and screamed in the key of F for Frantic. One of the boys raised a chair over his head and aimed to throw at me. I just looked straight at him and stood my ground. No chair hit me. Much to the student's despair, I didn't seem bothered by his language or his threatening chair.

Inside me of course, I thought about how easy it would be to fall if the chair hit me. As far as the tantrums and threats, I became quite good at using the intercom when needed. I always had a sense of angelic protection, and it came to me whenever I was in a scary place. It was that sense that allowed me to stand my ground and not show my students fear. My angels have protected me well throughout my life, and I knew they were not going to stop then.

Music classes continued, and by the second week we were on our way to learning lyrics and songs, along with some instrumentation for our PTA Christmas program. I was very proud of those students, and I knew I would miss them very much. The Christmas show was a big success.

I left my substitute teaching job at the end of December when the assignment was finished. I then began looking for another full-time music therapy job. I found one the following March. A Florida state-run hospital system, built to house mentally retarded (now identified as Intellectually Challenged) wards of the State, had finally been condemned. The State had to find placements for all clients who had lived in the state hospital. Some had lived only part of their lives in the hospital. However, many of the clients were hospitalized for their entire lives.

Florida had decided to fund a new concept: building ranch-style homes in clusters of three or four houses structurally placed in their own cul-de-sac. They were set up to hold eight children per house. They were known as ICFMRs (Intermediate Care Facilities for individuals with intellectual disabilities). The clients from the condemned hospital were going to live in home-like environments, and all clients were assigned their new group home placements. I was hired as the full-time music therapist for one of the clusters of group homes in the Orlando area. This cluster had three houses. It was really exciting to design the first music therapy treatment plan for such a new concept.

The majority of the clients were at the severe or profound levels of intellectual disability, mostly non-verbal, as well as quite medically involved. They were in wheelchairs or rolling lounge chairs. Many had a degree of paralysis. I designed music therapy sessions for all of the clients, which meant I had to haul my musical instruments and sound equipment between the three group homes. I found a pushcart I could handle on the paved walkways between each house. I always loved my music therapy jobs, so when physical demands arose, I used my creativity to adapt. I never let my disability stop me.

I was proud of my work, so I was so excited to share it with my mom during one of her visits to Florida. I took her to the group homes and gave her a grand tour of the facility. I introduced her to all of the clients. I will never forget my mom's reaction. She was very quiet and looked quite uncomfortable. At first, I thought she was tired after traveling for hours and had just arrived. However, when I finished my tour and gathered my things to go home for the evening, my mom said, "Dianne, how can you work with those kinds of clients? They can't even talk to you. Some have feeding tubes and tracheotomies to breath, so how do they know what you're doing with music therapy?" I replied, "Come with me."

I took her over to a group of clients that were gathered in a circle. Their wheelchairs were positioned for them to watch TV, but the TV wasn't on yet. My mom sat off to one side. I went to the closet that housed my equipment and grabbed my guitar. I came back to the circle, guitar in hand, and put a chair in the middle of the circle. I then announced, "Hey everybody, how about making some music with me?" I began to play and sing some of their favorite songs. The clients' faces lit up with smiles. Some made loud sounds, which was their way of singing, and flapped their arms in rhythm. I called out their names and brought them into the songs. The staff came and joined in, and we had ourselves a great sing-along. One of the nurses took a client's wheelchair to dance with that client. Everyone there could hear laughter and see the joy the clients felt, and I did too.

My mom sat there and smiled. I saw tears in her eyes, but being the strong-willed mom that I knew, she kept it together. I finished our therapy session saying, "Boy, you guys know how to make music! Let's do that again tomorrow." My mom and I said our good-byes for the day and left. Out in the parking lot, before we got into the car, my mom said, "Well, Dianne, you are meant to be here. I never dreamt you would work in a place like this, with these types of clients. It really takes a special kind of person, Honey to be able to work with them." I replied, "These clients are people, Mom. They have personalities, needs and wants, just like us. I see them as people that God made. In fact, I think they are the human Angels God made for us to care for. You and I both know that if you and Dad didn't fight to keep me as an infant, and had instead taken the advice of the female doctor at the teaching hospital, I would have been a ward of the State of Iowa. I would have been living in a hospital for crippled children, just like these clients. They didn't have parents that fought for them like I had, and still have. So really, Mom, your decision years ago made it possible for these clients to know me, and for me to share God's gift of music, which He gave me for them to have." Needless to say, we both had tears in our eyes as we got into the car.

While working at the group homes, I met some wonderful people. They were all of the same mindset; our clients were people who needed to be treated with dignity and respect. Unfortunately, the state-rum hospital system they all came from was not run on that philosophy. All of the group-home clients had lived most of their lifetimes inside a very institutional environment. It was a big undertaking for the State of Florida to create a *normalized setting,* and to introduce the clients to a dignified world. The transformation was amazing, and it was very rewarding for me to be a part of it.

I became very good friends with the staff recreational therapist Karen, who became one of the closest and dearest friends of my life. Our two training programs were similar, and although we didn't know each other before working together, we had both gotten our degrees from FSU. She was a very quiet and observant woman and one of the best listeners in the world. She was an incredible therapist, too, and the clients opened up, smiling during any contact with her. There was a collaborative team of various modalities on the staff, and I was really blessed to experience such a work environment. Working with Karen influenced me to become a more attentive and quiet observer. Karen made me a better music therapist. Having her as my close friend ended up being a huge gift from heaven above. How huge that heavenly gift ended up to be would reveal itself soon.

～

I WORKED for a year and a half at the ICFMR, and then received a call from the principal of the special school I had substituted for earlier. He said that his music teacher had retired, and he wanted me to start the new school year as the full-time music therapist. Let's just say, I got off the phone after saying, "YES!" I then created a very unique *happy dance.*

I loved that job and all the requirements that went with it. I even got the principal to have the school board finance ramps for all the portable classrooms, not just my portable. I loved most of the faculty, especially my friend Helen who was the art therapist there. She is still one of my closest friends today. I remember many of my past students; some with smiles and some with my head shaking and wondering how I managed those situations. I have many wonderful memories, and one in particular is very precious.

Within the school faculty, we all agreed upon certain students who were angels and certain students who were far from angelic—ones that some of the faculty members labeled the FCA (Future Convicts of America.). One boy stood out. He already had some experience with the law and juvenile detention. He was probably the toughest kid in the school. All of the students knew him as the King of Mean and they worked hard to avoid crossing his path. I didn't have very many classroom problems with him, because the principal had counseled me on his school record and his police record. I established my ground rules with him from the very beginning. That's not to say he didn't try to break those rules, but he and I came to a very good understanding. One day in my second year at the school, a new student was enrolled. He was in the King of Mean's classroom. Not surprisingly, the two of them decided to see who could keep the title of "king."

When the class came for their allotted music therapy class time, the new student began by yelling extremely colorful obscenities, along with making some threatening moves towards me. I turned on what I carefully called my *Hitler mode of classroom management* and just stared at him. I sternly walked toward him and told him to sit down. I kind of felt like a hero in a western movie. The new student didn't move toward me. He just looked at me. Somewhere from the chair to his left came a voice from the King of Mean that said, "You better not mess with Mrs. Wall, because she always wins!"

I had all I could do to stifle my laugh and keep a straight face. I never had another incident with that student, and the King of Mean and they became fast friends. I set up a separate and special music therapy time just for the two of them to come and play the drums and any other instruments they wanted to play. Their classroom teacher supported the plan, on the stipulation they earned the privilege by good classroom behavior. I was proud to say they earned most of those sessions. When it came time for them to graduate and move on to high school, they both came and said, "Music is our favorite class in school. We're going to miss you Mrs. Wall." I said smiling through tears, "I'm going to miss you guys, too,"

Another memorable moment was when I was chosen by the school's faculty as their Teacher of the Year. I represented our school at the Annual County Teacher of the Year Awards Ceremony. I was so honored to represent our school that year, that I didn't care I wasn't chosen County Teacher of the Year. I really loved being part of that faculty, and loved my music therapy program I had designed. I felt that was my dream music therapy job for years to come. That was my plan. However, God had a different plan. During my fifth year at the school, I had to take a leave of absence early in February. I had the worst case of morning sickness ever, and I was going to be a MOM! The year was 1986.

~

MY HEAD WAS SPINNING with a mix of emotions: happy and excited that I was pregnant but also scared. I remembered what doctors had always thought—the risk of pregnancy would be very high for me. I knew that it would be physically difficult for my body to carry the extra weight of a full-term baby, but my faith told me that I would have the strength to face the risks. I also felt sad to leave my dream music therapy job.

Dennis was scared for me, too. He knew the risk that pregnancy created for me, but he loved me enough to face that risk with me. We had always shared our faith together, so now we were relying on that bond of faith.

I also dreaded telling my parents of our happy news for fear of how my mother would react. I knew she would be scared. I also thought she'd be mad at me for taking such a high risk. I was right to dread the call. The first words out of her mouth when I told her were, "Oh sh**!" Of course she followed that up by saying, "It'll be okay, Honey. I will be praying to St. Anne, the Blessed Mother's mother, who I prayed to while I was pregnant with you." I replied, "Thanks, Mom. Let's just hope those women in heaven didn't hear you say sh** first!" We both laughed.

My sister Maureen who was living at home with Mom and Dad at the time of my call, later told me that when Mom got off the phone the color drained from her face and she looked terrified. Maureen always says it reminded her of Sally Field's reaction to her daughter's pregnancy in the movie, *Steel Magnolias*.

I was also worried about my pregnancy, because Dennis and I had made a major decision the prior year ahead. In August of 1985, we decided that he should open his own law firm, which he did in September 1985. We had discussed all the pros and cons and decided the time was right for starting his own practice. Since I had a good job in the county school system with good benefits, and we had no children the time, we both felt it was a good plan. Although we had talked about wanting children, we had tried for years with no success. So after seven years, we thought it probably wasn't meant to be.

I laugh at us now, since that was exactly what my parents thought when they decided to adopt. But then God's plan for their bigger family took over their lives. In the same way, our lives were living out God's plan for us. Even with all the emotions inside my head, I knew it was going to be all right.

I left my music therapy position in February 1986 on a disability leave of absence, thinking that I could come back to my job after the baby was born. My due date was August 31st. As it turned out, Dennis's legal secretary was pregnant as well and due the very end of February. She was planning on training her replacement the last two weeks of that month, once Dennis had time to find the temporary secretary. Well, God laughed at that plan, too.

Dennis's secretary went into labor the first weekend of February, and Dennis didn't have a temporary secretary hired yet. So, no sooner had I left my full-time music therapy job than I had to help Dennis as his part-time legal secretary—after my morning sickness hours. I was trained by Dennis, using all of the notes his legal secretary left for training. I never thought that as a music therapist that I would become a legal secretary.

Electric typewriters were the main piece of office equipment used by legal secretaries in the 1980's. I was happy I had taken a typing class in high school, which I barely got a C in. Typing bored me. Hitting typewriter keys wasn't as much fun as hitting piano keys. During typing class, I would hit the keys to certain rhythms and make fun of it. However, the teacher would occasionally stand behind me while looking and listening to my *rhythms*. "Listen McTaggart, your typewriter's keyboard isn't black-and-white with eighty-eight keys, so knock it off." I was amazed he knew the piano had eighty-eight keys.

Like I said, I was lucky I got out of his class with a C. I will always give him credit though. I knew that my arms would have a very difficult time reaching a typewriter, so at the beginning of the semester, I met with the teacher and explained my disability to him. Out of the thirty typewriters he had for his class, only four were electric and available to the students. He always had students rotate and take turns on the electric typewriters. However, for me he suggested I stay on the electric ones for the entire semester. He accepted my disability with the can-do attitude that I was so accustomed to. No wonder he was perturbed with my typing *rhythms*! Thanks to his good and patient typing instruction, I learned what I needed to know about typing. And with only a C grade, I helped Dennis keep his new law office open so he and I could become parents.

About a month after starting my legal secretary job, Dennis found a good temporary secretary. I could only work about four hours a day, and even then, some days I was too sick to drive to the office in downtown Orlando. By April of that year, I was into my second trimester, so I was starting to feel good again. My OB-GYN doctors followed me carefully, since they had labeled me a high-risk patient. My pregnancy was smooth going during that second trimester, which was a very good thing.

During the mid-1980's, typewriters were starting to be phased out of corporate offices, including law offices, and replaced with a new technology called word processing. That required legal secretaries to be trained on computers. While working in the school system, I had been generally introduced to Macintosh computers, but the legal world used a different processing system manufactured by Wang. Fortunately, the temporary legal secretary who Dennis had hired had some training in Wang. Dennis needed me to purchase the computer system for the office and be trained by Wang sales. I was then ready to get the extra training the temporary legal secretary offered. Much to my surprise, I discovered I loved computer work and word-processing. I became very computer literate, and I learned all kinds of equipment needs for a legal office. I went from being a music therapist to Dennis's office manager. However, the computer bug bit me enough to make me want to learn how to apply the technology to music. I had to put that desire aside though, since the baby was taking up my energy and was definitely my top priority.

THE COUNTDOWN HAD BEGUN for my August 31 due date. My third trimester began, and it was demanding strength from my body that was very hard to find. I could still walk, but my body had started to retain lots of water. I had only gained fifteen extra pounds, but for my body it felt like fifty extra pounds. I bought my very first cane at the end of July, after my doctor ordered me to. I knew he was right. I knew I needed it for safety and balance. I hated using a cane, something I never thought I would need. However, I knew reality was telling me I needed the help.

I had to accept my disability in a way I had never had to before. Driving was too dangerous. I could no longer reach the pedals or the steering wheel because of my tummy area. I could not work for Dennis anymore, and I was mostly homebound. My dear mother-in-law Edna came over to the house every day during the month of August. The threat of me falling due to the extra weight I was carrying was a reality that Dennis and I had to face. With Edna helping me, I could rest more and felt more secure.

My friend Karen continued to play a big part in my life, especially during my pregnancy. Karen had gone through one year of nurses' training at FSU before she switched to recreational therapy, so I knew she had a strong stomach. Dennis and I had talked about Lamaze classes, and the need for Dennis to be my Lamaze partner, but he reminded me how much he hated hospitals. So, we thought it was a good idea to ask Karen to be my official Lamaze partner and be my coach in the delivery room. That way, Dennis could feel free to leave the room if the needles and "hospital stuff" started making him uneasy. I told him that I would have enough to worry about delivering a baby, without having to worry if he was going to get queasy. He agreed. Karen became my Lamaze partner. She drove me to all the Lamaze classes, and we worked on our breathing and all the great things women learn from the Lamaze technique of birthing. I felt so blessed with Karen's friendship.

My little sister Maureen was getting married in Iowa on August 2. I was so sure I could fly up and attend, as well as sing for her wedding. However, the doctor would not allow me to travel being so close to delivery. Walking and getting up from chairs, as well as toilets, were getting to be next to near impossible without assistance. I knew it was important to stay home, but I so wanted to celebrate with my family and sing for my little sister's big day.

I knew there was a way to use technology to record something to send up to my sister. I was lucky that I was a regular volunteer cantor at my church, because I was able to arrange to have the music director come to my house and accompany me singing what Maureen had chosen for me to sing. Thanks to technology, I was able to record it.

My church's sound equipment man had the knowledge and equipment to mix the recording to make it sound like I was singing live at the wedding. I sent it up to be played at the wedding. Technology made me feel like I was part of my sister's big day. That was the next best thing for me being there in person, and in turn, my sister had the wedding videotaped so that I could see it. It wasn't as easy as today's technology, but it got the job done.

When I look back, I realize I used technology as an adaption to participate in life. I was ahead of the *digitalized virtual world*. I was going to be at my sister's wedding my way, eight months pregnant. I invoked my inner belief that I could find a way to do what I set out to do, because "somebody told me I could."

That is how I faced my pregnancy—believing I could carry my baby to a full term and deliver naturally, without a Caesarean section, although several doctors thought it would be wise to schedule one. However, my lead doctor in the OB-GYN group thought if I wanted to try for natural birth, I should at least try.

My August 31 due date came and went. I was waddling around with my cane very carefully. I stayed inside the house with the air conditioning on high, since late August and early September in Florida are not the most comfortable months for a nine-months-pregnant woman. Any mother-to-be can tell you, having to go to the bathroom almost every ten minutes during the last four weeks of pregnancy is very normal but also very tiring. Sleep is constantly interrupted due to the baby laying low and on top of the bladder. All pregnant women have to get up a hundred times to go potty each night. Sleep is a nonexistent gift you wish for but seldom get enough of.

One night, shortly before my birthday on September 8th, I got up to go potty. As I got out of bed my legs couldn't hold me. I fell landing on my knees first and then on my belly. Dennis woke up with my scream for help. He rushed to pick me up off the floor. I was so frightened that the fall had hurt the baby. However, as I often did, I brushed myself off and checked to see if I could feel the baby move or show any signs of distress. Thank God, everything felt normal. Although I was still shaken up. I noticed I hadn't even scraped my knees, and I whispered aloud, "Thank you God for always protecting me."

Dennis helped me to the bathroom and then got me back into bed. I lay there rubbing my belly while talking to my baby and thought, "Okay, kid, you gotta be tough, 'cause your mom just took you on your first carnival ride." I finally felt the baby move, just as it did every night, so I thanked God again for having my fall be a softer one compared to many of my other falls. I calmed myself down by saying my rosary to the Blessed Mother and somehow fell asleep.

The day following the fall I struggled to walk more than before. Dennis and Edna were watching me very carefully. I could see they were worried. I was hoping I would go into labor on my birthday. I thought since September 8th is the Blessed Mother's birthday, and mine too, it would be so cool if the baby could share our birthdays with us. However, God's *divine blueprint* was not mine.

The day after my birthday Dennis drove me to my scheduled checkup. The doctor checked me out, and all my vitals were good. The baby had a good heartbeat and was moving normally. However, when I told the doctor about my most recent fall, he was very concerned. Dennis spoke up and told the doctor just how hard it was for me to get around. Dennis had a way of telling the doctors the whole truth and nothing but the truth, in a way I never did.

Dennis and the doctor both looked at me and the doctor said, "Okay, Dianne, I am calling the hospital now to get you admitted, and we are going to induce labor. We can't take a chance on another fall, so don't argue." The doctor had my number for sure. I didn't want to argue though, because I was so tired of feeling like a beached whale. Dennis drove me directly to the hospital, and I made a quick call to my parents to let them know. This time, my mom said, "God's with you, Honey, and you will be alright."

4

My pregnancy had been followed by a well-respected OB-GYN group of about six to eight doctors. One of the younger doctors in the group followed me the majority of the time throughout the nine months. However, one of the group's senior doctors would see me occasionally because I was a high-risk pregnancy. During the nine months of group rotation, I was seen only once by the youngest and most recently hired doctor but he was very aware of the risk that my labor and delivery would be for my body. He told me the hospital maternity ward had one birthing chair, and he recommended that I use it. He said the chair positioning used the benefit of gravity, and that would make the pushing ability much easier for me. I thought that was a great idea, and I made a note to myself that I would request the chair.

By 1:30 in the afternoon on the ninth of September, I was hooked up to a Pitocin drip (the drug used for inducing labor). I successfully responded to the drip by dilating to ten centimeters within an hour, though labor pains did not really begin until later. My request for a birthing chair was denied by the senior OB-GYN in charge over the younger doctor. This senior doctor had followed throughout most all three trimesters more than any other doctor in the practice group. When I objected to being denied use of the chair, the staff told me it was already in use, and they only had one. I didn't believe them then, and I still don't believe them to this day—but I lost that fight.

The person assigned to me who I thought was my anesthesiologist (a doctor), and who I later learned was actually an anesthetist (a nurse), came in after labor pains had increased in late afternoon. He said he would give me an epidural so I wouldn't have to be in so much pain. I informed him that I wanted natural labor.

I also explained to him that with my severe scoliosis, I felt it would be dangerous to put an epidural needle in my back. I told him I had enough problems with my back, and that a slip of the needle in the wrong place was not a risk I needed or wanted. I told him that I was not a stranger to pain and I knew I could handle the pain without his epidural.

After a lengthy discussion, he took my request seriously. I have no doubt that he later noted in my file that, in his opinion, I was a non-compliant patient. I was not a stranger to that label, and I practiced my self-advocacy proudly. Dennis and my friend Karen were at my side. The anesthetist looked over to the two of them in hopes that they would convince me of his recommendation. However, they looked at each other, smiled, and just shrugged their shoulders as if to say, "You heard her, Doc!" I knew what risks I was willing to take, and Karen understood and respected me for that.

My intense labor pains came later that night. By 10:30 p.m. I had pushed as hard as I could. By 11:00 p.m. the baby had crowned, and the nurse could see its head full of dark hair. However, doctors told me not to push because the baby's shoulders were too wide for a natural birth. They said they needed to do a C-section.

So from 11:05 p.m. on, I screamed at anyone who would listen, and held my baby inside. Those Lamaze breathing exercises were definitely a help, and Karen and I had some fun with a technique that we named the "Dizzy Gillespie maneuver." Dizzy would play his trumpet with the puffiest cheeks ever. Being the musician that I am, I told Karen that we would name the puffy-cheek breathing after Dizzy.

Karen was constantly calling me Dizzy during that holding time, and in between screaming and swearing, we would laugh heartily.

It took the doctor and nurse birthing team forty minutes to get me into the operating room. They told Dennis, Karen and me that it was due to a previous delivery complication. I remember screaming at the anesthetist to hurry up, because I was going to push no matter what they told me to do. The last thing I remember was looking at the clock. It was ten minutes after midnight, September 10, when I was finally put out of my misery.

I remember the time so well, because I kept watching the big clock all day in my delivery room. When I was wheeled into the operating room, I spotted the clock right away. I wanted to remember how long it would be before I saw my baby. The doctors and nurses told me I should be able to see my baby pretty fast, once the C-section was done and I was in the recovery room. However, that was not the case.

After I was wheeled into the operating room, the first thing I remember was a dream that I was walking in a gray tunnel and I saw my father-in-law who had died of cancer five years before. He was off to my right, smiling at me. He had on his favorite plaid pants with a shirt that didn't match, which was so him. He looked really healthy and happy, which is not how he looked the last time I had seen him.

Although I could hear and understand while he spoke to me,

his mouth didn't move. He told me, "You know that it isn't your time yet, and you have to go back." I smiled back at him and said, "I know." Neither of our mouths moved, yet we were talking to each other. I just remember how big his smile was. I was so happy to see him.

I really wanted to stay, because it was such a nice place to be. It was a calm and peaceful feeling. I felt such a love that words cannot describe. I also remember a total absence of fear. Although it was a soft gray around us, I saw a bright light in the distance.

Dad and I just stood staring and smiling at each other, and then in a blink, I was watching the anesthetist fighting with another doctor who I didn't know. I later learned from Karen, who was in the recovery room with me at that time while Dennis and Edna had gone to the nursery with the baby, that the breathing tube was removed from me, and the doctor told Karen to wake me up. She told me that no matter how hard she tried, I wouldn't wake up, because she knew I was dead. She had to convince the doctor to come over and see for himself that I was dead.

I had already turned gray and was not breathing, with my mouth open and my tongue out. Karen said she knew I was dead because she had training with cadavers during her first year of nursing school.

I also learned years later that many PPS patients react to anesthesia. One group of anesthesias are neuromuscular blocking agents, and the drug used for my C-section was definitely from that family of drugs. Neuromuscular blocking agents turn off the nerves that send messages to the muscles, and in my case, all the muscles that worked my heart and lungs shut down. Medically stated, I went into total respiratory failure and cardiac arrest.

I saw both doctors stand behind me at the head of my bed,

and yet I was watching them as if I was watching a movie. A blue mask (Ambu bag) was over my face, and that the anesthetist was manually pumping air into me. He and the other doctor were fighting about giving me another test cc of epinephrine and putting the breathing tube back down my throat. The unfamiliar doctor, who was clearly in charge of my anesthetist, yelled back at the anesthetist and said, "No, you can't give her another test cc of epi. You already tried a test cc that didn't work. You have already put this body into shock, so you can pump that Ambu bag 'til your arm falls off!"

I must have become conscious after that "movie," because the next thing I remember was opening my eyes and realizing I couldn't catch my breath. I saw a nurse at the foot of my bed. The anesthetist was at my side squeezing something blue that covered my nose and mouth. I could not breath when I tried to, and yet my breathing was happening in a very weird rhythm. It finally dawned on me that I couldn't breathe on my own. The doctor I had seen earlier in the "movie," the one I did not recognize, explained to me that the anesthetist was assisting my breathing, and that I needed to allow him to keep assisting for just a little while longer.

At that point, I was sure that he was the one in charge. I later learned that he was indeed in charge, and the hospital's Director of Anesthesiology. The OB-GYN doctor who delivered my baby called him in immediately when the delivery team saw my body shutting down and called a "code-blue."

Thanks to the experience of September 10, 1986, I definitely know the difference between an anesthetist and an anesthesiologist.

The nurse I had spotted at the foot of my bed started to talk to me. She told me how brave I was. She said that I had to keep fighting to breathe, because I had a beautiful little girl waiting for me in the nursery. I thought, "Oh, I had a girl." I looked at the clock and saw it was 2:20 in the morning. I kept staring at the clock with such disbelief. How could it be that time? I thought to myself, "Where have you been, Dianne, for the last 2 hours?"

The doctors finally allowed Dennis into the recovery room, and he came to my bedside and held my hand. I remember seeing him and not being able to speak to him, because my mouth was covered with the pump. I can honestly say that there have been MANY times Dennis would have appreciated my inability to speak, but this wasn't one of them. I could see he was scared and exhausted.

He told me that he had held our little Katie, the name we both agreed for naming a little girl. He said she was beautiful like me and very strong and healthy, weighing seven pounds and three ounces. After a while, the doctor tested my breathing capacity, by slightly lifting the blue pump off my mouth. The minute he did, I looked at Dennis and tried to tell him to say a Hail Mary.

He got it. Dennis starting praying it out loud. When he finished with it, I tried to say, "Again," and I kept signaling to repeat it over and over. I just remember the two of us praying the Hail Mary together repeatedly until the doctor in charge gave the okay to remove the pump from my mouth and nose. My fear level was slowly lowering, and my fight to keep breathing was no longer such a fight. I eventually started breathing on my own, although it felt like when you can't catch your breath. I just kept pushing my lungs as well as I could, until my normal breathing pattern came back. I was totally exhausted, but I couldn't wait to see my little girl Katie.

Two nurses wheeled me out of the recovery room, and Dennis and Edna were able to go home, knowing I was going to be okay. I reassured them all I was more than okay, and said my good-bye to Dennis. Karen stayed, with her camera in hand to catch every memory she could. Then the nurses asked if I wanted to stop by the nursery on the way to my room. My face told them, "What in God's name do you think I want to do?"

They smiled at me, and we waited in the hallway while one of the nurses went into the nursery. She returned with my Katie wrapped up in a blanket with a little pink knitted hat on. Karen's camera was clicking away.

I couldn't believe how beautiful and precious Katie was. I had seen lots of movies with scenes of mothers seeing their babies for the first time, but no movie could ever prepare me for the feelings that swept over me in that moment.

When Katie's eyes looked at me, I felt that she knew I was her mom. Since I had been through hours of fighting in my battle to live, I didn't have the strength to hold her, but the nurse held Katie close enough for me to give my little girl her mother's first kiss. I'm happy to say that, thanks to Karen, I have a beautiful picture of that moment.

They took Katie back into the nursery and then continued transporting me to my room. I said goodbye to Karen in the hallway and told her to go home and try to sleep. I told her I could never thank her enough for being there and being my friend and angel. I remember her tears and her nod while saying goodbye. At that moment, I had not yet learned that it was Karen who saved my life that night by telling the doctor I was dead, but I knew she was there during my battle. I knew she was more than a friend to me. She was much more like a sister, and I thanked God for her as she left to go home.

Once the nurses got me settled in the room, I looked up at the clock in the room and saw it was after 6:00 AM. I was finally aware of my exhaustion. I still had lots of wires on me monitoring my heart and lungs, along with an IV. When they left and shut my door, I was out like a light. However, before I fell asleep, I said a huge thank you prayer to God for such a beautiful baby girl. I also thought to myself, "Wow, I did it," even though my mom and doctors said I shouldn't. I believed I could, because somebody along the way said "You can do it, Dianne, but it will be your way." I knew that Somebody was God the Father, Son and Holy Spirit. I also knew that my way was really Our way together, as it had been since the day I was born.

PART IV

LIFE WITH POST-POLIO SYNDROME

5

Motherhood was a true adventure and challenge. My creative adapting skills were definitely used and appreciated. I figured out ways of picking Katie up, holding her, bathing her, and everything else that goes into being a mom. Dennis was a huge help, but he also had to go to work. Thankfully, my parents flew down to stay for a week once I was released from the hospital, where I remained for a week after the delivery.

Edna took over once my parents left, and she came over to the house every day. Eventually, it was Katie's idea to name her Nanny Nana. Whenever my mom visited, she was known as Grandma. Katie named them both at her second birthday party. She just pointed to them and declared their names, along with naming my dad Pop-Pop.

Without Nanny Nana's help, my body could not have done it as well as it did. I was also blessed with an amazing child who knew intuitively that I needed help. I called her my little rhesus monkey. Every morning I would go to pick her up out of the crib and she would grab ahold of my nightgown with her hands and arms and hang on, allowing me to hang on to her as well as my arms could. As Dr. Ponseti had told the young doctors he taught years ago, "Dianne will figure out how to hold a baby and do things her way."

Karen was still a big part of our lives, and Katie knew her as Aunt Karen. Although she lived almost an hour away from where we lived, she would show up for all birthdays and holidays, and shower Katie with gifts. Katie was Karen's little sweetie, and as always, Karen was a dear friend to me and the best ear a young mom could have.

By the time Katie was two years old, I felt my arms and legs were weaker than ever before. At first, I put it down to not sleeping as well due to listening for Katie at night. We had a one-story, split-plan house. Katie's room was clear across the house, so I slept lighter in order to hear her. However, my back, neck, and torso had pain that I had never felt before. Dennis wanted me to get checked out by the Orlando orthopedic doctor who had been recommended to me by Dr. Ponseti. He knew Iowa doctoring was out of the question due to me living in Florida. I reluctantly made an appointment.

Although he wasn't like Dr. Ponseti, he was a very good doctor. He was older than Dr. Ponseti, which meant that he had lived through and practiced medicine through the polio years. Time was marching on, and there were many younger, practicing doctors who did not have any experience with people who had polio. My new doctor had gotten my history from the teaching hospital. I remember he told me that I was really blessed (his word, not mine) being a patient of Dr. Ponseti. He said that God's Angels must have picked him for me, because I had had the best doctor ever. I got to know my new doctor and his ways and learned that we both shared the same Catholic faith. After my first visit to his office, he asked me to make the next appointment for thirty days from then. He also requested that I bring Katie to the next exam. He wanted to see how I picked her up and all of my creative ways of mothering.

The following month I went to my scheduled appointment with Katie and Dennis at my side. Katie and I showed the doctor our ways of picking up, holding, feeding, bathing, and how we otherwise helped each other. The doctor quietly observed and smiled as he watched. When we were finished answering his questions and doing our demonstrations of creative living, he wanted to talk to me about his observations, so Dennis took Katie outside to the waiting area.

He explained that my new weakness and difficulties were due to a recently discovered medical condition, called Post-Polio Syndrome (PPS). This was 1988. During the previous year, due to all the medical reports of polio survivors experiencing new weakness, the National Institute of Neurological Disorders and Stroke conducted a U.S. Health Institute Survey. My doctor explained that he and his fellow practitioners were still waiting for the publication of the results. However, he also explained that many practitioners were finding that within fifteen to thirty years of the polio virus striking a person, there is a pronounced weakness and severe fatigue in the patient that had not been present before.

I took all his information in. It was his medical opinion that I was clearly a PPS patient. I had never heard of PPS before that day. He recommended I join the local Orlando PPS support group, and he gave me some contact information. The doctor then smiled at me and patted my hand saying, "Dianne, that support group could use a person like you. You have the outlook on life that some of the other polio survivors might not have, and so I urge you to find out more about them and join up." I told him I'd consider it, but I wanted to know if he had a treatment plan for my PPS.

He told me that there was no cure or magic pills, but that

each case was different. He said that since I had been quite medically stable for the past 30 years, he felt I could learn from the support group how to maintain the strength that I had. He assured me that I could always call his office if I needed him.

I left the doctor's office feeling like I had just fallen and had to figure out how I was going to get myself up. On the ride home, Dennis and I spoke a bit about what the doctor had to say, but I didn't really want to talk much about it. Why couldn't the doctor just give me a prescription for the pain in my neck and back and send me home? I wanted to cry, but I knew it would upset Dennis and Katie and the drive home wouldn't be very safe or pleasant. Plus, my head was spinning with all the information I had just learned, and it didn't fit into my past experience with Dr. Ponseti. I had always beat the odds and figured out how to do whatever I wanted to do. With PPS, it sounded like my independent streak was just run over by a dump-truck. It was that day that I began using a new phrase to describe the fatigue and pain I had started experiencing—my dump-truck days.

That evening when we had put Katie to bed, Dennis and I sat down and discussed PPS and what I thought my future would be. As always, Dennis listened patiently and let me cry. However, when I was finished with my pity party, he encouraged me to go and find that support group. He told me he believed in me and that I would learn all there was about PPS. He felt the group was probably a good first place to start, learning from other people with polio. So, the next day I called the contact information I had been given, and I found out when the next group meeting was. It was only a twenty-five minute drive from our house, and it was being held on a Saturday afternoon. There was nothing to stop me from going, except my own fear.

∼

I chose not to deal with the fear for about two years, even though I knew through faith that fear never comes from God, it was just easier to live one day at a time. Life was full and I made sure I stayed busy raising Katie. We had moved into a new house not long after I first learned about PPS, so I was busy settling into our new home as well. Dennis was very busy as a sole practitioner, and I was busy being a mom.

I pushed through my fatigue days and just kept going. I told myself that I wasn't going to decline like other polio people with PPS. I read up on the medical condition and knew that it varied in everyone who had it. I convinced myself to stick to my "can do" attitude. It had gotten me through everything in my life, so I was sure God was with me and in total agreement that I had to keep going.

One day in 1989, Katie was helping me pick up the house so it would be nice when Dennis got home from work. I had picked up a pile of newspapers, and I went out to the garage to put them in the recycling bin. While I was stepping up the one step to come back into the house, my left leg lightly bumped the door frame and down I fell. I yelled to Katie to get help. She was only three years old, but I told her to roll the kitchen chair over to the telephone that was on the wall, in a little kitchen desk area. She was crying and scared because I was scared too, but I had to be strong for her and not show my pain. Fortunately for me, she was an incredibly smart three year old who knew her numbers all the way to a hundred by then. I had her pick up the phone, and told her what numbers to push to call our neighbor Jeannette across the street. I couldn't physically get back into the house. So from the doorway while still on the garage floor, I told Katie to tell Jeannette that I had fallen and to ask if she could come over and help.

Jeannette and I had become very good friends since moving into the neighborhood. We had become such good friends that we had already exchanged house keys with each other for emergencies. She came right over and picked me up and put me in a kitchen chair. I knew I was in trouble because I couldn't walk on my leg at all.

Jeannette called Dennis, and he came home from work. He took me to a neighborhood emergency clinic where they examined me and took X-rays. They found I had fractured my kneecap and needed to be seen by an orthopedic doctor as soon as possible.

My orthopedic doctor was out of town, so I made appointment with another one I had heard about for the next day. After the new doctor examined me and took my history, he read me the riot act.

The new doctor could tell I had the potential to be a hardheaded patient. Who, me?

He told me to keep my leg in the cast for eight weeks without ever bending my leg. He also said that if I didn't do what he ordered, he would meet me in surgery to put a pin in my kneecap.

I listened to his every word, like the model compliant patient I decided to be. I had never broken a bone before, even with all my stunts. At least I was familiar with a cast, but I was thrilled that this one was removable, and worn on the outside of my pants. This cast was a gift; I could scratch my leg if it itched!

I followed the doctor's orders perfectly (well...almost), and my four-week checkup and X-rays showed that my kneecap was slowly healing. It did completely heal in eight weeks. On my last visit, the doctor had me walk up and down his hallway. He kept saying to do it again and again. It reminded me of my Dr. Ponseti appointments when I would be asked to show the young student doctors how I walked.

However, this doctor finally said to me, "How can you do that? How can you walk on your left leg? You do not have the muscles to support your knee, and yet you are walking. I have never seen anything like this before." I told him how Dr. Ponseti always called me his puzzle child, and I guess that my walking was part of the puzzle. This doctor smiled and said, "Well, if the great Dr. Ponseti couldn't figure the puzzle out, I'm not going to question it. It's clear that whatever your body is doing, it's doing it right for you."

No doctor had ever told me that before, that I don't have the muscle that actually supports the knee. I guess it explained many of my falls. Dr. Ponseti always made me feel like I was put together in a special way, and in the way that worked for me, but he never said I didn't have muscle or that my spine was in the shape of a letter S. He would always put it in a positive way. I always left my appointments with Dr. Ponseti knowing that I could do anything, but in my way. So, I told this new doctor that even if the muscle doesn't respond and is totally atrophied, my walking works for me and it's my way.

Of course, I always knew, and still do, that it's God's way. He designed it just for me, and it works.

I did like watching this doctor's face while he watched me walk. It has always been fun to show doctors possibilities, especially when they were taught that the body couldn't do impossible things without the right parts. I have learned since those first days of PPS that for the sake of explaining things to patients, doctors would say, "You don't have the muscles," but that really isn't medically accurate.

We were born with all the same muscles as everybody else, but when polio struck it went to our brainstem and zapped the nervous system which controls all muscles. Polio prevented my brain from sending messages to the nerves wrapped around the brainstem. Those nerves travel to all parts of the body and attach their motor neurons to the muscles, which tell the muscles what to do. Polio "fried" many of my motor neurons, making my muscles atrophy. Polio damaged my entire nervous system, which affects much more than my muscles, but my brain adapted to the changes, and I have learned how to live life quite fully.

The fall that fractured my kneecap was a lightbulb moment for me. I hardly tapped the doorway the day I fell, yet my body broke so easily. Osteoporosis, a thinning of bones, had set in due to the lack of bearing weight on my left leg, which I've always referred to as my bad leg. I knew falling was never going to be quite the same for me as before. I knew that if I ever fell down on my knees again, and I landed on them in many of my falls, my kneecap would break again. I was only thirty-six years old, but my body was aging much quicker than other thirty-six year-olds.

The fear of PPS came back to me. I knew I couldn't wait to learn more about it. I knew I had to go to the local PPS support group and learn how to live with this new challenge I was facing.

After a few months of getting my strength back following the cast, I looked up the next meeting of the support group and went. I had never been around many polio people before. They called themselves polio survivors, not victims. I had never thought of myself as a victim, but I had never thought of myself as a survivor either. I soon adopted the survivor title for myself too. There were over twenty of us there at the first meeting. Most were older than I was, but a few were only four or five years older than me.

We all introduced ourselves and told our polio stories. I was amazed at the many variations of how the virus changed their lives.

When it came to me, I said I had been born with polio. There was a gasp from many of the members, and the leader spoke up and asked me to explain what that meant. None of them had ever heard of being born with polio. I explained as briefly as I could, and I answered many questions from the members.

When the meeting ended, the president of the group came up to me and asked if I would stay for the board meeting after this general meeting. I told her that I would consider staying for the next board meeting, but I had to go home and think about all the stories I had heard, as well as read the information packet I had been given that day. I had peeked at the information packet during the meeting and was surprised at the various resources available to me. I left the group that day feeling so blessed. I was blessed to have met these people. We were all so unique, yet all so the same.

I did join the board of the PPS support group and was active for several years. However, as the members aged, and life's demands on all of us grew, the group meetings ended. I learned so much from their advice. They advised for me to get my first mobility scooter in order to conserve my energy. They also advised me to get a minivan with a lift for the scooter. I had never thought I would need a scooter. After watching so many of them use their mobility devices, even though many of them could still walk, I thought why not me, first too. However, I waited until 1993 to get my scooter, minivan and lift.

The PPS support group changed me and my life. I wasn't as afraid of my body's decline. My fear diminished, and my new PPS friends showed me life can still be full. We were all survivors.

6

Ever since the early years of our marriage in the 1980's, and up to the time I became pregnant with Katie, I had always volunteered at church playing my guitar and singing for one of the weekend Masses. Poor Dennis got used to always sitting alone for Mass. He didn't like it much, but he knew that music was such a big part of me. He knew I was answering a call to share God's musical gift, and he respected me for that. I first started volunteering for the 12:30 p.m. Sunday Mass. After a year of playing and singing for the 12:30 p.m. Mass, the Pastor recruited me to take over the Saturday 5:00 p.m. Mass each weekend, as well as being the volunteer choir director for that Mass.

In 1990, when the full-time music director was leaving her post, I applied for the job and got it. Dennis knew that, even though I was needed at his office, I missed my music. So, as he had always done, he supported my decision to take the job. I kept up with office-managing and payroll for his office one day each week, even while I took on the full-time church position.

Since I knew the parish music, I thought the job would be easy for me. I was in for a big surprise. Being the full-time music director meant weekly staff meetings and I went from handling one Mass, to handling five Masses each weekend. I had to sing at all funerals, weddings and special sacraments, as well as plan and coordinate all High-Holy times of the liturgical year, like Christmas and Easter. I had great support from the director of religious education, Mindy. She helped me in many ways, but the best way was her ability to listen to me. She, too, was pushed by the demands of her church position and understood the frustrations I felt. To this day, she and I are still extremely close friends.

Between my office manager role and my music director role, not to mention my wife and mother roles, my life had become a little too full. I knew after nearly two years of being the music director, I knew it was too much.

I left the job in the spring of 1992 and I never regretted taking the job, nor leaving it. I was able to go back to the joy of being a volunteer and kept my love of music. Most importantly, I was able to see Dennis and Katie more. Katie had started elementary school in 1991, so there were many more parental demands that needed my attention. Without the full-time director job, I finally had the time to be home more for my family.

My PPS support group had taught me the philosophy of "conserve to preserve" and why that was the best mantra for any polio survivor. But I certainly wasn't following that philosophy. I could feel my weakness and fatigue level increasing, and yet I kept telling myself I was fine and strong.

I was working several days at the office with Dennis while Katie was in school. Nanny Nana picked Katie up at the bus stop on the days I worked. I was experiencing more pain in my neck and back with more weakness in my arms and legs. Sitting at a computer, plus doing many other office duties like filing, was getting to be painful.

As polio survivors have confirmed many times over, our

bodies gave us many warning signs through the years that our Type-A personalities chose to ignore. I was living like I had been taught: "You can do anything you want to do, but you'll do it your way." Although I would still take occasional falls while pushing my limits, I was always able to heal and not break bones, particularly my left kneecap. So, I just kept living life to the fullest.

It was a busy time in the early 1990's, raising Katie and doing all the things I loved. I was also dealing with a heavy sadness after learning my brother Kevin's secret. He lived in Chicago and worked for an airline, so flying down to visit a couple times a year was easy for him. In February 1987, he came down to visit. I was excited to see him and introduce him to his new niece for the first time. While Kevin was visiting, Dennis told us to go out and have a relaxing supper, while he babysat Katie.

While we were at the restaurant, Kevin said, "I don't know how to tell you this, but I have to. I am HIV-positive and have been for a year now."

I was his closest sibling, and he needed to tell someone in the family. But he waited to tell me, since I had been pregnant with Katie when he received his diagnosis and had given birth to her just six months prior. He didn't want me to tell anyone else. He especially didn't want me to tell our parents.

We were from a family who beat medical odds all the time, so we both tried to stay positive. However, back in the 1980's, HIV-positive was an early death sentence that progressed into full blown AIDS. I became his confidante, his health surrogate, and the executor of his will.

Dennis helped me through the many years of watching my brother suffer. I finally convinced Kevin to tell our other siblings in 1992. I felt they could help Kevin break the news to Mom and Dad. Since Kevin lived in Chicago, and all of my other siblings still lived in Iowa, I knew I lived too far away and couldn't be present when Kevin finally got up the courage to tell our parents his news. Kevin agreed with me that Mom and Dad would need to have time to brace themselves. He knew that our parents needed time to make some memories with him, as I had been doing since 1987.

I flew to and from Chicago many times during Kevin's years of medical treatments, and I helped Kevin navigate his way through his medical maze. Toward the end, in late 1994 and spring of 1995, my older brother Pat and my younger sister Maureen each took a turn for a week at a time, staying by Kevin's side. I had been with Kevin in the fall of 1994, and February of 1995, so Pat and Maureen's visits helped me have a break from traveling. We were very lucky that Kevin had arranged for hospice care to be at his apartment, so we didn't have to be in a hospital during his last months.

Dennis could see how much it took physically and emotionally for me to balance my life with him and Katie in Florida, while also supporting my brother in Chicago. He was very worried about me. Dennis knew if I got too physically drained I would start to fall especially with all the traveling between Orlando and Chicago.

That was the last thing he wanted me to have to go through. I also knew he was right. I knew everything would fall on his shoulders if I was injured in a fall. However, Dennis supported me in every way possible. I know that, without his support and love, I could never have been strong enough to help Kevin face death. He was my closest brother, and we were very connected.

Toward the end of Kevin's battle, during the second week of May 1995, I flew up to Chicago to be with him. The doctors thought he only had a few weeks left. Our mother was also there. I was expecting to find Kevin incoherent and weak in bed when I arrived, but he was quite aware and even joking around. He had refused morphine until the very last week of his life, because he wanted to be in control of his faculties. During my stay I had the time to make some very fond memories with him and our mom. We laughed a lot. We prayed a lot. Most of all—we loved a lot.

One afternoon, while Kevin was resting in bed, I went to sit next to him. Kevin and I shared a wicked strain of our family humor, so I said to him, "So you haven't said anything about my new hair highlights. You have to admit, it's a big change from my dark hair." Kevin looked right at me with a straight face and said, "Well, Honey, I was going to say you look a little processed!" We both just broke out laughing, and we could feel our hearts lift from the sadness of having to say goodbye soon. So then I asked him, "Okay smarty, it looks like you're closer to heaven than I am right now, so tell me this: what is the secret to life?" Not missing a beat, Kevin replied, "Good hair products."

Moments like those kept me strong during that very difficult time. He hung on for another month, and kept beating the medical odds, so I flew home.

It was a roller-coaster ride for Dennis and Katie. We had to arrange childcare for Katie, because Nanny Nana couldn't watch Katie constantly as it became too exhausting for her. Somehow Dennis and I found childcare coverage, and Dennis and Katie continued their sacrificing and held down the fort at home.

A week after I returned back home from Chicago after my visit in May, I received a phone call from my dad. He said Kevin had just called him crying, and Dad said, "Honey, Kevin told me he doesn't think he can die without your love, and he is sure he doesn't have long." Hearing my father's words broke my heart. Dennis helped me pack, and the next day I was on the plane back to Chicago.

There was really no predicting when Kevin would die because he would rally and then stabilize. Kevin was still hanging on after another ten days in Chicago, when his doctor said he might last several more weeks. I had to return to my husband and little girl. They certainly hadn't seen much of me during the many months of travel. It was very hard on Katie, who was only nine years old and being passed from babysitter to babysitter. So, I kissed my brother goodbye while he was in and out of consciousness, and told him I'd be back, and caught a flight home.

My brother died two days later. It was June, 1995.

~

DURING THE MONTHS after my brother's death, I continued to ignore the PPS group's "conserve to preserve" advice. I was the Executor of Kevin's estate, which meant that I had to clear out all of his apartment and his life in Chicago after arranging his funeral in Iowa. My brother Pat and my sister Maureen drove with me to Chicago after Kevin's funeral. I could not have done it without them.

Fortunately, I had booked a moving company before Kevin had died. It was a company that specialized in helping families dealing with death by AIDS. They put me on their calendar and told me to call as soon as my brother died. They knew first-hand we needed help during a tragic time. AIDS was a major epidemic in Chicago during the late 1980's and 1990's. So many Chicago people were angels to me and my family. I felt like Kevin was directing it all from heaven.

I was exhausted much of the time, but as always, Dennis, Katie and my dear mother-in-law helped me through it. By the end of that year, life had settled down a bit. However, my friend and neighbor, Jeannette was diagnosed with an advanced stage of renal cell cancer. I was about to lose another person I loved.

Jeannette's husband Ernie called hospice to help. I visited as much as possible. Jeannette died in February 1996.

Since I was familiar with the "business" of death, I arranged Jeannette's funeral and cremation. I even sang her favorite songs at her funeral Mass. One of those favorite songs was about life-long friendship. I had always promised her that I would sing it at her funeral. It's the kind of song that you need to listen to with a tissue in your hand.

I had to practice getting through it without needing a tissue. Jeannette had always had a wonderful sense of humor. To steel myself the day of her funeral, I remembered the precious time when we laughed our heads off at the last luncheon we shared at our favorite restaurant.

While sitting at our table, I told Jeannette she should feel very honored that I took her out to lunch. After all, just that very morning, I had shaved my ankles in her honor! I am someone who HATES shaving her legs. I told her since I always wore jeans, people would only see my ankles, so why bother with the rest of my legs. She let out the biggest laugh and said she was so tickled that I had shaved them, especially for her. We were both laughing so hard and loud, we had tears running down our faces. Our poor waitress just shook her head. I know her manager wanted us to hurry up and finish our meals. We gave the girl a nice tip as we left, still tear-streaked and laughing. With that memory, I sang for my friend's funeral and fulfilled my promise with her favorite friendship song.

By March of 1996, my father got very sick. He and my mother lived in Arizona for the winter months, so Dennis, Katie and I flew out to see him. It was April by then, and when we arrived, he only had one day at the house with us before we had to take him to see his doctor. I drove him to the hospital immediately after his doctor's appointment. The doctor said it was time for the ICU, since Dad's heart was down to thirty per cent capacity, and his lungs were down to twenty per cent when. We were glad to be there with Mom during this time, and we all prayed for Dad's fighting spirit to kick in.

However, he didn't have enough strength to fight. The hospital staff got him comfortable and somewhat stable. We all hoped he could make it back home in a week or two, but we knew we couldn't stay that long. Once again, I said goodbye to someone I loved very much, knowing it would probably be my last time. His last words to me were, "I am so very proud of you, Dianne. I love you." My father died three weeks later in the same hospital that I had driven him to.

We all flew up to Iowa for Dad's funeral in June. I was the family member that arranged the funeral Mass and worked with the priest. Dad always said he wanted me to sing at his funeral. I had managed to sing one song at Kevin's the year before, but only one. However, I knew I would never get through singing for Dad, so I arranged to find a little recording studio in my hometown and recorded all the songs for Dad's Mass. The church music director played the recordings during the funeral, and I was able to be with my family. Death was something I was intimately familiar with, but it never felt good.

Traveling was getting to be very taxing on me, but I knew the drill. I had great assistance from the airport staff most of the time. However, the biggest support I had was from Dennis. He watched me slowly wear myself out, and yet he always supported me in every possible way. He was the one and only person who could get it through my thick Irish head that, if I kept going at this pace, he'd be the one planning *my* funeral. I knew he was right.

～

MY LIFE WENT BACK to a routine of raising Katie through her elementary and middle school years. I still worked part-time at

Dennis's office and volunteered for the church music ministry. Katie's school years were racing by so fast and were full of activities. Our little girl was getting older, soon to become a teenager.

Around 1998, I felt a calling to record a CD of some of my favorite hymns. Kevin had once told me that, because he and I shared the gift of music in our hearts, he knew that music was a big part of my soul. He and Dad had always wanted me to record. With both Kevin and Dad in heaven, I really felt like they were setting up the possibility of making my recording dream become a reality. However, trying to find a recording studio that I could afford was the biggest challenge of all. Just when I thought I had found a studio in Winter Park, Florida (only twenty minutes away from our home), the owner explained how much time and money it would take to record a group of songs for an entire CD. He explained that it was more realistic to just record one song, due to cost. I understood the prices he was quoting, and I knew what he said was true. I began to think maybe my dream should just stay in my heart and head. I wondered if God was trying to tell me something. I knew I needed some time to think and to pray on this recording dream of mine.

I had not been feeling too well for many months and finally went to my gynecologist to find out what was going on with my aging body. She told me it was time to have a complete hysterectomy, since I had already gone through four dilation and curettage (D&C), procedures in the past. D&Cs are done to remove tissue from a woman's uterus. I had a bad case of endometriosis, which makes tissue build up inside and outside the uterus. I knew that it could become cancerous if not removed. The doctor explained that even if I had another D&C, my problems would not go away, and my risk of cancer would increase. So, I scheduled the surgery and put my recording dream back on the shelf. It would take two to three months, at least, to recuperate fully, so I had time to think and pray.

I made it through the surgery without problems and felt very blessed. The same anesthesiologist who saved my life twelve years before when I gave birth to Katie was able to be the anesthesiologist for this surgery as well. He always told me he would be available to help me through future surgeries, and he had given me his personal home number in case the need ever arose. Being the head of Anesthesiology, he had learned my complicated body very well the night of my fateful birthing experience, and he knew I would probably need his services again. I did need him for four of my previous D&Cs. Knowing that he was well aware of possible PPS complications, he always made me feel safe as I faced many surgeries.

As I explained earlier, the polio virus struck my brainstem, which killed off much of my nervous system. Good anesthesiologists know that a PPS diagnosis tells them to carefully watch a major cranial nerve called the Vagus nerve. It is the longest nerve in the body, and interacts with the heart, lungs and digestive tract. If an anesthesiologist uses the wrong drug to anesthetize a PPS patient, the heart and lungs of the PPS patient can shut down. There are many anesthesia medications, so picking the correct one is a challenge. That is exactly what happened to me giving birth to Katie—the wrong medication was chosen. However, since the head of Anesthesiology was the one called into that emergency, he knew exactly how to safely anesthetize me.

Once healed from my surgery, I was kept busy helping Dennis at the office. Katie's softball and band activities kept us all hopping. No matter how busy our lives were, Dennis encouraged me to keep trying to find a way to record my CD. I hadn't given up on recording, but the time that was given to me to step back and heal allowed me to keep believing in my dream while surrendering it to God. I reminded myself that His timing is not my timing.

We had allotted a certain amount of money to do the recording project, so I just had to find the right musicians and studio within that budget. I shared my dream of recording with a choir member I had gotten close to while I was choir director at the church. She said that her daughter knew a professional musician who might be able to help. Luckily, her daughter's friend did know of a fabulous pianist named Harry, who graduated from Juilliard. He also worked part-time at a recording studio that a local theme park used. After meeting with Harry, I explained my dream project, as well as my budget. He agreed to do it.

He told me that he could use the studio for personal projects, but it had to be in between the big projects scheduled during the days. He scheduled our sessions on evenings and weekends. I was so thrilled and in total awe of his talent. It was a dream getting access to such a professional studio. It took us a year to complete, mostly because of arranging our sessions in between the studio's full schedule of business.

There was a bit of a roadblock after the very first evening recording session. It was a super good session, and we recorded *Forever Friends.* It took many hours to lay down all the instrumental tracks. The instrumental tracks then had to be coordinated with my vocal track. That was the last step to do. I was at the studio from 6:00 p.m. until 1:00 a.m. By the time I got home at 2:00 a.m. I couldn't fall asleep. I think I was singing in my head all night long. I was on cloud nine, with a big sense of accomplishment. My dream was coming true. I knew getting out of bed that morning after having been awake all night I had to be extra careful not to fall. I was supposed to go back into the studio the following night.

While letting my dog outside that afternoon, I fell on my

back porch. It was solid cement. I knew when I landed that I had fractured my left kneecap again, for the second time. I still had my old cast from 10 years ago, so I put it on to keep my leg straight and protected. Once again, I was at the doctor's office for an X-ray. I was lucky the same orthopedic doctor was still practicing, and he told me that I healed well before, so I could do it again.

Since I couldn't drive, I couldn't record for over two months. I just had to be very careful and give my leg time to heal. It did heal completely, and I started recording again with Harry in the same studio. We finished recording the project in December 1999.

My friend Karen asked if she could come to watch and listen on the last night of recording. Of course, I said yes. I had one final song to complete, a song about where we go after death. Karen didn't know what song I was recording, but I did. I knew this song was a very powerful one. The lyrics spoke of faith in knowing that, when we die, we will be welcomed back into God's Love.

Karen had been diagnosed with renal cell cancer a year earlier, in 1998. Her prognosis was not good. It was very difficult for her to tell me her diagnosis. Karen knew what I was thinking when she told me she had renal cell cancer. It was the same cancer that my friend Jeannette died of in 1996.

Renal cell cancer is rather rare as cancers go. How could two of my closest friends have the same cancer with the same dire prognosis? How could the woman who saved my life now be facing death? The emotions that flooded me were overwhelming. Thinking that life wasn't fair didn't cover what I felt. However, I had to be strong for Karen. I vowed I would be there for her as much as I could.

Throughout our years of friendship, Karen always supported my musical endeavors. She came to most of my concerts and attended several of my singing gigs. I tried to think of my last recording session as just another time my friend was supporting my music. As I watched her through the window of the recording booth, I saw that she had been ravaged by repeated surgeries and chemo.

As I sang the song, I saw the smile on her face looking at me as if she knew she was going home. There were several times during the recording when I needed to stop and gather up my strength to finish. Neither Karen nor I shed a single tear the entire recording session.

I remember on one of the session breaks, I told Karen I had to go to the bathroom, but I had to get my purse first. She told me she would be happy to watch it for me while I went. However, I said, "Karen Honey, my purse hides my secret plastic container. I need to sneak my plastic storage container into the bathroom, so that Harry doesn't see me taking it in with me." Karen just looked at me with a very puzzled look, and I said, "I have mastered how to pee standing up! The toilet is way too low for me to ever get up from if I ever got down on it. Squatting is too dangerous because I will end up going down for sure. I have mastered a position where I catch my urine in the container while standing over the toilet, and then I dump it in the toilet when I'm done. Brilliant, huh? I mean really, Karen, I had to think of some way to keep from yelling at Harry that I was stuck on the can!"

We both laughed until we had tears in our eyes. I knew my humor was the medicine our hearts needed to complete the session.

When Harry gave me the cue that the song was complete, I took my headphones off and walked to where Karen was sitting. We walked out of the studio together and smiled at each other. This was the mask we each wore to stay strong for each other. As we hugged goodbye, I said, "Thank you for making this night the best ever Karen." She had tears in her eyes, and I didn't want us to end the evening that way, so I said, "Now remember me next time you need to put leftovers away in a plastic container!" We walked to our cars laughing.

Due to mixing and mastering the final tracks, it took until late March 2000 before the final master CD was complete. I received publishers' copyright permissions for all of the songs I recorded. Since there were several different composers, I had to contact the publishers that represented each song. I titled the CD, *Touched By The Light*. Finally, I found a local company who mass produced and packaged my CDs. It was quite an education for me.

I wrote one of the songs on the CD, and my sister Maureen helped with the lyrics. It was a song about our brother Kevin. We both agreed that we were called to write the song, just like I was called to record an entire CD. With all the hard work completed, I felt a huge sigh of relief and a sense of accomplishment. My dream came true, and I sold a good number of them.

I set up my own music business, where I gave inspirational talks and sang songs from my CD. For each gig I was hired to do, I had to have "roadies" cart the heavy (sixty pound) PA system, along with the two heavy speakers (twenty-five pounds each) to the venue. Dennis and Katie were always my helping "roadies." Once the equipment was at the venue, I set up the cables and microphone myself. Once again, I was pushing the limits of my body, and I could feel I was getting weaker. However, I didn't want to stop doing what I loved to do so much, which was to sing. I was using my scooter more, thinking that it would help conserve my energy. I was also using my cane more to walk. But even trying to support my body with mobility aids, I knew I was taking a big risk.

I had developed a good relationship with Dr. Mitchell Freed after meeting him in 1996 while being evaluated at the Orlando

PPS Clinic. That was the clinic my PPS support group encouraged me to go for evaluation. I was examined by an inter-disciplinary team of doctors, physical-occupational therapists and orthotic specialists (specialists trained in diagnosing braces, as well as various support devices). The PPS clinic confirmed what I had been told years ago, when I was in my thirties. After being examined for hours that day, I reflected on my body's decline during the previous ten years. I listened to all the specialists' summaries of their examination findings and knew that I had to take it seriously, or the next ten years would be the end of Dianne as I had always been.

Years following my PPS clinic evaluation, I went to Dr. Freed for treatment of my PPS symptoms. He was a physiatrist, which is a rehabilitation specialist. He was a specialist in PPS, MS, and many other physical disabilities, as well as sports injuries. He taught me how to live with PPS and how to make wiser decisions to conserve and preserve my strength. He always said that our goal was to maintain as much as we can, for as long as we can. I always agreed with that goal. However, deep inside me, there was this voice that kept saying "Yeah, Dianne, but you're not going to lose!" As time went on, I knew that voice was wrong.

~

KATIE STARTED high school in 2001. She was active in band and was also in our church's theater group. In 1999, we had changed parishes to a much larger one than before. The new parish, St. Stephen Catholic Community, had many more programs for middle school and high school students. The church was also much closer to our house, so many of Katie's school friends were members there as well.

I volunteered at our new parish to teach religious education classes for Katie's age group. I stayed away from volunteering in music. I knew it would be nice for a change to sit at Mass alongside Dennis and Katie. And it was nice. I also knew that I needed a break from a music ministry.

That went well for about six months, until the pastor, Father John, found out I was a trained musician and a past church music director. He wanted me to talk to the music director at our new parish and to consider joining the choir. He said he knew I had plenty of experience cantoring, so he wanted me to consider that as well. I told him I could never be one of their many cantors since their music area had very steep steps—ones I could never make. Plus, the cantor stand steps didn't have any railings. I never have been able to do steps that are over four to five inches in height without railings. It's a huge risk. I finally said, "Father John, thanks for the vote of confidence, but bottom line, cantoring would be way too risky for me." He replied, "Let me work on that. I know the guy in charge over there."

Dennis knew before I did that music would draw me back. I joined the music ministry and became one of the many cantors leading the singing for various Masses. Father John had steps made up to the cantor stand with a railing included. He made sure they were only four inches in height— ones he knew I could make. When I did not cantor, I sang in the choir. The choir chairs were hard for me to get up from, so I would bring my own cushion to raise me up about three inches. The cushion enabled me to rise much easier. Before long, Father John had the parish carpenter make special risers for my chair, so I no longer had to use my cushion. Throughout my life, adaptive changes have been provided for my accessibility issues. I have always believed that God gave me my musical gift, so I knew God would provide a way for His gift to be shared—a gift I have always loved sharing for His glory, not mine. I grew to love the music ministry and our new parish.

Life was still busy with family and work and volunteering.

Two big changes came in 2002. First, I received news that Karen had lost her battle with cancer. It hurt so much to know I couldn't save her life like she did mine, but I sure wished I could have.

She died the day before her birthday, July 14.

I was not able to visit her while she was at home with hospice, due to accessibility issues I had developed with my changing PPS body. I stayed informed and kept in contact with her family as much as they could handle. Karen's mother had developed stage-four lung cancer in 2001, so her father and her brother had home hospice care for both of them at Karen's house. It was a very sad time for me. Karen's wishes were not to have a funeral. She was always a very private person. Many of our co-workers who worked with Karen and me at the group home got together several months after Karen's death. We had a celebration of life in her honor. I knew Karen was one of God's Angels on earth, and now she was home with God's Love. I also knew that love doesn't die. I would have her in my heart forever —she was one of my *Forever Friends*.

The second big change in 2002 was my mother, who was then eighty years old, by then decided to move from Arizona to Florida. She had lived alone in Arizona for six years after my father's death, and she knew it was time to be around family.

I had three siblings in Iowa who wanted her to come move back there, but she decided she didn't want the cold winters.

I knew Mom wasn't in the best of health, but she was independent and still driving, or so I thought. She decided on an assisted-living apartment about ten minutes away from our house.

I thought it would be great to have Mom here. She would be able to see Katie more. Katie only saw her grandparents once a year while growing up. I thought how wonderful it would be having Mom participate in family activities, like attending

Katie's band concerts and theater productions. It would be a chance for me and Mom to have special time together—to shop, or go to movies, or eat out. It was something I hadn't had since leaving Iowa nearly thirty years prior.

However, those plans ended within a few months of her arrival. Mom's health was very bad, and she was in and out of the hospital repeatedly. Once again, Dennis watched me take responsibility for family. I became Mom's medical advocate. He also watched with deep concern the toll it took on my PPS symptoms. I was getting weaker, but I just kept pushing through.

In August 2004, our home was hit hard with Hurricane Charlie. My mother was safe at her assisted living apartment, although very scared. I was thankful that she was not alone, and her center was equipped to take care of elderly people during a storm. Our house still had a roof after the storm went through, but we had much damage in the yard. We also lost power for over a week. Luckily, Mom's place got power restored within two days. My mother-in-law was safe in her condo, and she also regained power after three days. The roads were blocked for several days, so we could not get to either mother.

We did manage to see and check up on them once roads were safe. It was a rough hurricane season then. Only two weeks after Charlie hit, we got another hurricane. My mother-in-law decided to go stay with her daughter, who lived more in the center of the state and not in the direct path of the storm. We got my Mom on a plane early, up to my sister's place in Iowa.

Right after Hurricane Charlie hit us, Dennis and I had to get our septic system completely redone, since the storm took down a huge tree that pulled the system out of the yard. Dennis agreed to drive me up to Iowa once the septic work was completed, with only a day or two to spare before the second storm hit. He and Katie dropped me off in Iowa, then the two of them turned around and drove back to Florida, driving through the storm itself. Dennis wanted to get back to protect the house, and Katie was hoping to go back to school.

It was a very scary time for all of us, but even after a third hurricane followed the second one, we all made it through safely. My Mom was still in and out of the hospital and rehab centers. She had become very medically involved. My older sister Colleen moved from Iowa to Florida, after all the hurricanes and tried to take care of Mom. The two of them moved into a house together. However, Colleen saw within a few short months that Mom needed more medical assistance than we could provide. In the Spring of 2005, we had Mom move into an assisted living center, one that included continued care if it was ever medically necessary. Colleen moved back to Iowa. Mom's new assisted living center was only fifteen minutes from my home. It allowed me to visit her easily and be able to transport her to frequent doctors' appointments.

During the time Mom lived here in Florida, Katie graduated from high school in 2005, was accepted to a nearby university, and started her college degree. Dennis and I were going to be empty nesters!

Also in 2005, my mother-in-law decided to move to be near her daughter, who lived about an hour-and-a-half away from Orlando. Nanny Nana and I were very close, and she watched how much time and effort it took from me taking care of my mom's health needs. She also knew that she was at the point in her life where she was going to need some help, too. Since she never wanted to be a burden to me and Dennis, moving to where her daughter lived made the most sense to her. She was a real stinker about it, too—she never told us until her move was completely settled. We were very shocked by her decision, but we always respected what she chose. I always knew she loved me very much, so I think she decided taking care of two moms would probably put me in the nursing home before either of them.

Nanny Nana was such a rock for me. She was my Florida mom, and the one I needed the most after Katie's birth. It hurt us to see her move.

2005 was such a busy time and filled with so much change. Three months after Nanny Nana's move, Dennis was diagnosed with prostate cancer.

We were both scared, but Dennis was strong. He even drove himself, all alone, to all of his forty-one radiation treatments. He never once complained. Since Dennis always hated doctoring, he said it was good I had so much medical experience going to doctors as a kid since I could help him navigate through the cancer treatments. However, I have to say that, for a guy who hated doctoring so much, he went through that scare amazingly strong. I was very proud of him.

Then came 2006, and Dennis had to deal with medical issues that arose from the radiation treatments. Once again, he was tough. No body goes through that many radiation treatments and comes back normal. It takes its toll in one degree or another. He took it one day at a time, and so did I.

My mom was a medical marvel, beating all her doctor's expectations. However, she continued to be in and out of the hospital. I was by her side as much as I could be. While being so active, my PPS mantra, "conserve to preserve," was again being ignored. I could feel it more each day.

In March 2006, Nanny Nana died. It was a very big shock for us, and I took it pretty hard. We had a funeral for her at our parish. Yes, I once again planned another loved one's funeral. Nanny Nana was such a huge part of our lives. I knew I would be eternally grateful for her love and life, and I knew I would forever miss her.

~

KATIE'S COLLEGE YEARS, 2005-2009, went by super fast. I was going to Dr. Freed much more often with new weakness in my neck and torso. My fatigue was very pronounced. I had started to fall more often, too. My body was rebelling, and I couldn't do what I had always done. I was using my scooter every time I had to leave the house, and I was never without a cane when walking was required.

I was blessed with a home health aide. My mom actually hired her in 2003 for herself. In fact, Mom realized how much she had begun to rely on me, so she talked me into hiring an aide to help me with laundry and grocery shopping once a week. My aide became a big help in giving me time to practice conserving and preserving. My tendency to push through still had big control over me, but Dennis would remind me to listen to my body and to ask for help.

All post-polio survivors will tell you their physiatrists must rule out any possible health issues before deciding PPS is the cause for their new fatigue and weakness. In my case, around the year 2000, I was diagnosed with low thyroid. That diagnosis explained my new lack of muscle strength and fatigue. Fortunately, it was controlled with medication. However, my fatigue during Katie's college years was definitely new PPS symptoms brought on by me living as a Type-A personality. "Conserve to preserve" was more often "shop til you drop!"

Ironically, being my mother's medical advocate, I kept pushing my limits and ignoring my self-care. My mother's physical decline was increasing, and her heart was getting weaker. She had also developed vascular dementia, which was increasing. She continued to be in and out of the hospital on a regular basis. After she had a heart attack and a stroke, Mom was finally moved to the medical care unit of her assisted living center. Our aide took Mom to most of her outside specialists' visits, plus occasional shopping trips, getting her out of the assisted living center once a week. That allowed me time to rest more.

In 2007, I finally asked Dr. Freed if I should stop working for Dennis and get evaluated for disability. That was the first time I had ever cried in front of him. It felt like I was giving up. It didn't fit my philosophy of life. I thought that I could do it all but do it my way. I had worked up to the age of fifty-seven, but I didn't have the physical strength to continue.

Holding my head up while filing was getting to be impossible. I continued singing at banquets and giving talks to clubs and organizations, but it was getting very hard to hold my microphone. I knew I was in trouble when I found it hard to sing.

I submitted my disability claim for evaluation, and within three months of the review my claim was accepted. Many people have to wait years and are often rejected the first time they file their claim. When I read the letter sent to me from Social Security, it informed me that I was rated a seven, out of a one to seven scale, with a rating of one meaning minimal disability subject to frequent review. That meant, due to my physical disability, they would never have to review my case again.

The Board of Disability knew I would never get any better than I was at the time I made my claim. In fact, my progress would steadily get worse. That was a shock to my system. I logically knew that it was the right decision to quit working, but I couldn't help but feel like I was a quitter. However, since my health insurance premiums had increased too much for us to afford them, I was very grateful for my acceptance and how fast it was processed.

Throughout my entire life, I had always been rated as high risk by health insurance companies. That rating was made due to my pre-existing issues. My insurance premiums were always higher than for someone my age who did not have similar pre-existing issues. Dennis was a cancer survivor now, but still working, and his premiums were steadily going up each year as well. At least with disability, I would have some insurance, which I learned was Medicare. I have to admit, I loved watching the medical billing staff's faces, as I filled out insurance information. They would look at me and say, "Medicare? You look really young for sixty-five." Of course as the years have gone on, it's not as much fun filling out the doctor's insurance forms.

Katie graduated from college in 2009. She didn't really know what she wanted to do for a living, but with a B.A. in Psychology, she was open to many different possibilities. It was after the Great Recession of 2008, so finding a job was hard. She moved back home and kept plugging away and submitting her resume.

I was kept busy with my mom, who was failing quite steadily. However, our aide helped to transport her for outings with me. Unfortunately, most of these outings were to doctors' offices. Mom had become wheelchair bound.

My mom had her own scooter when she first moved to Florida. I helped her get a scooter lift on the back of her car, so she could use her scooter when shopping and going out to places. We used to meet at the malls, since we each had our own scooters. The looks we would get from people were pretty priceless. We were both speed demons and loved to drag race. Malls were spacious enough that we could drag safely. I can't remember which one of us thought to race each other first. I wouldn't be surprised if it was my mom who suggested it first. Neither one of us could move very fast in our daily living, so the thrill and freedom of a *scooter drag race* was just what we both needed. She always won because her scooter had more power than mine. The best part of our RESPONSIBLE drag racing was that it always ended with a perfect dose of laughter.

~

KATIE FOUND a full-time job in the spring of 2010. She had moved into her own apartment only thirty minutes away, with her best friend from high school. I had begun my constant gratitude prayers many months before, thanking God for finding Katie the best job possible and in His perfect time. Katie moved out on Holy Thursday, got a job offer the next day on Good Friday, and started her job the Monday after Easter. I knew it was God's perfect blueprint.

As I have grown older, I have been practicing an "attitude of gratitude" more and more. With a chronic health challenge with no cure, I have found that surrendering to each new moment makes living less challenging. I also know that God decided to bless me with many opportunities for patience. His timing is not my timing, but His timing is always perfect. We are all given plenty of patience-practicing moments. With my Type-A personality, a type that many of my fellow polio survivors share, I know I will be practicing patience for many years to come.

By May of 2010, my mother had declined so much that, during a medical procedure in the hospital which required her to be awake during a catheterization, she screamed at the doctors and nurses to stop everything and let her die. Since she was still medically competent, they stopped the procedure as she requested. A nurse came out to inform me, "Your mom demanded we stop the procedure. It was just too painful for her. Your mother's wishes were noted by several doctors, as well as myself and two other nurses. We had to honor her request." I said, "Thank you for doing that." She replied, "If it was my mother, I would do everything possible to make her comfortable and honor her by respecting her wishes."

I went to my mother's bedside and said, "Tell me what you want me to do for you, Mom." She looked so frail and frightened lying there. Her fighting spirit was no longer in her eyes. "I never want to come back to the hospital, and I never want another needle stuck in me ever again." She said, "Honey, just let me die without all this hospital stuff." I nodded and said, "I promise you that you will never have to come back to any hospital ever again or be pricked with anymore needles. You know I will stick up for you no matter what."

I then left the hospital and our aide stayed with my mom until the doctor could clear her for release. I drove over to the assisted living facility. I went straight to the doctor's office in their clinic. I met with the doctor and explained what had happened at the hospital. I told her that the hospital staff working on my mother's case had documented Mom's wishes. The clinic's doctor looked at me and said, "When the treatment is worse than the disease, it is time. I recommend you consider palliative care, and I will get you some contact information. You have been a very good daughter, Dianne, and I understand what you must be feeling." She smiled and walked away. I sat there remembering talking to my siblings earlier that day. We discussed whether Mom really knew what she had agreed to when this invasive catheterization was explained to her. I tried to explain as much as I could to Mom, but her dementia was on and off. Mom thought she understood so she agreed to have it done. My brother and sisters and I were all on the same page. How many more procedures would really give Mom better quality of life? They were the ones who pushed me to call for hospice care, and now Mom's doctor thought it was the best thing for Mom as well. I called hospice that very day.

After my mother was back in the nursing facility, hospice came and evaluated her. Nobody, including me, ever told her who was evaluating her. However, I knew my mom was a pretty sharp cookie and probably figured it out. I also knew that she was the best *queen of denial* when it came to her own reality, so I played the game and hospice did, too. Their evaluation stated my mother clearly met the medical threshold for palliative care.

They agreed she was a medical marvel and they determined she might live quite awhile, so they planned to re-evaluate her every six months. They saw she had a very strong will to live. I agreed with everything they said and signed the papers as mother's medical surrogate.

A few days later I asked my aide to take Mom out shopping to her favorite store. It was only a block away from the assisted living facility. It was the drugstore that Mom used to drive her scooter to. I was still exhausted from the hospital-hospice sequence of events, so I could not join them. Even though Mom didn't like being in a wheelchair, she loved getting "sprung from the joint," as she put it.

The aide pushed her up and down the aisles and just let her browse and point to things along the way. My mother asked her to stop at the display section of "intimate" male and female items. Mom asked to see a box of condoms, and the aide tried to tell her that she probably didn't need, or even know what that particular item was. However, my mom, who was very hard of hearing, quite loudly said, "Oh I know what they are used for. They're kind of like a glove for men. You better grab me a box, because we have a wandering fella at night who gets horny!"

Everyone within earshot lost it, laughing their heads off. I share that story with you, because whenever I would feel sad for what my mom was living through, I would recall that drugstore moment and laugh my head off. It was another trait that I inherited from her: a very strong spirit of living with humor.

In the first week of June, just a few weeks after her drugstore shopping spree, Mom called me on the phone after supper. She said, "Call Pat up in Elkader. Tell him to find me an apartment or a house to live in. My vacation here in Florida has been way too long. I have to go home, Honey." She couldn't tell me how long she had been here, but she knew she had to go home to Iowa.

I told her, "I can't do that, because you're too sick to travel, Mom." She then asked, "How long have I been here with you in Florida?" I said, "Almost eight years." She gasped for air and said, "Why can't I remember that? Oh Dianne, what have I put you through?" I reassured her as well as I could and responded, "Mom, you only put me through love."

My mom died five days later. The hospice doctor said that Mom probably had a bladder infection that went septic. She died within a day of being diagnosed with a fever. I felt it was good that she didn't have to suffer long with the infection, but losing her wasn't easy. At least she got her wish to go home to Iowa.

~

AFTER MY MOTHER'S DEATH, I settled into life without so many doctor's appointments and trips to emergency rooms and hospitals. I took advantage of my aide's help, and tried to put the "conserve to preserve" mantra at the top of my priority list. However, I had the opportunity to be a music director for a community theater. I went to Dr. Freed for a checkup and asked him what he thought. As always, he listened patiently. He suggested it might be too demanding on my body. I reassured him that I would pace myself and told him I really wanted to get involved in the project. He reminded me that I would need to rest between rehearsals and to stop when I felt fatigue hitting me. He also knew me. Stubbornness was a wide streak in me, but so was my musical passion. He advised me of the medical consequences and said, "Be careful!"

Whenever Dr. Freed wanted me to REALLY listen and follow his advice, he would put it to me in a question. Like when I didn't want to accept his advice on getting a ramp-van for my scooter, instead of transporting my scooter with a manual lift as

I had been doing for years. I was experiencing pain in my left shoulder joint, that was very deformed from polio, and Dr. Freed had been treating it for a while.

On this occasion, he put his question to me this way, "Dianne, do you want to have the use of your left arm ten years from now?" I immediately thought to myself, am I going to fall apart that much in ten years? Didn't he mean twenty years? I mean after all, I was only in my fifties. But I looked at him as he patiently smiled at me, and I knew he was right. I smiled back at him and replied, "Yes. I guess I'm going to get a ramp-van."

The theater project was six months long, and I was very happy I accomplished the musical challenge. As for the physical demands, it was hard. In hindsight, it was too much. However, as I had done all of my life, I ignored the pain and loved the challenge. I went back to participating in my church choir, and cantoring occasionally. I was noticing more fatigue and difficulty holding my head up while singing. My back muscles were beginning to spasm when I stood to sing, which cantoring required. I knew my body was talking to me, telling me to stop. I cut back on cantoring and sang in the choir while sitting. Our director Betty knew that it was up to me to tell her when I could or could not participate. With her great support, I still felt a part of my musical life.

I stayed active by helping Dennis with some business matters, as well as mentoring some students who wanted to learn guitar, piano or singing. They kept me young, and I loved presenting music to them in a fun way. In 2013, I had a great opportunity to work with one of my dear friends from my church choir— Diane with only one "n". She was a professional stage performer who had been on Broadway for four years. She and I had a brainchild of an idea to do a "broadway revue" for our pastor's Fiftieth Jubilee celebrating his ordination to the priesthood. It was yet another musical opportunity to perform and to co-direct with Diane.

We became partners in "rhyme and crime," and we had so much fun getting fellow choir members to participate. We kept the show a secret from Father John—well only to a degree. He knew the choir was practicing for his celebration, but he had no idea it was going to be a two-hour revue. I did pace myself for that, and I really felt a sense of accomplishment. I also knew that vocally I was hitting sixty years old that year, and there were not going to be many more years that I would still sound like myself. Even with a normal body, vocal ranges change and breath control becomes a big issue.

I was thrilled to get the opportunity to create and direct. Working with a talent like Diane was also a dream come true for me. She had worked with top-notch show-biz personalities. I felt honored to co-direct with her. As she and I agreed, we put on a helluva good show....oops, it was in church...it was a heck of a good show.

In 2014, Dennis and I decided to get a brand new puppy after our sweet Schnauzer died at the end of 2013. Everyone told us we were crazy for wanting to go through house-breaking and all, but we had our hearts set on a Westie (short for West Highland Terrier). Our first dog was a Westie named Mickey, and we had him eighteen years. We also adopted a two-year old Westie named Zoe, when Mickey was about fifteen years old. After both our Westies were gone, we rescued another Westie named MacGregor who was about, five. He came from a puppy mill rescue and was very sick, and we had to be put him down after only a couple of months. We decided we wanted a brand-spankin' new puppy. No more rescue dogs, and this would be our last puppy. On September 7, 2014, we traveled across the State of Florida and picked up our dog. We gave him an Irish name, Seamus, (pronounced 'Shay-mus' in English).

He was a lively young pup and full of energy. After having him a month, we heeded the warnings of getting a puppy. We knew that Seamus was so active that he was a threat to my safety. We nick-named him Tigger, due to his jumping, and White Lightning, because he ran like the wind. I had a good friend from church who was in a wheelchair and had a service dog, so I asked him if he knew of a good dog trainer. Luckily, he did. We lined up training as soon as we could. Seamus quickly learned the commands of sit, down and stay. However, I, myself, needed training in consistency.

One afternoon in late November, I returned from a dentist appointment around two o'clock in the afternoon. I had skipped lunch earlier, so I decided to make myself a smoothie. Seamus loved Greek yogurt. When I got that out of the refrigerator to put in my smoothie, he ran over to me. That was the last thing I remember.

The next thing I knew, I woke up around 8:00 p.m. in ICU at the hospital. Dennis later told me that I had called him on the phone to tell him I had fallen and to come inside from his backyard office. When he got inside the house, he found me on the floor propped up against my recliner, looking kind of dazed. He said I asked him to make me a smoothie. I do not remember anything, so I can only tell you that Dennis called Dr. Freed's office and told his nurse that I had fallen and was talking funny. Dr. Freed got on the line right away and told Dennis to immediately call for an ambulance. The best we can figure, Seamus had knocked me down in the kitchen and I hit my head on the hard laminate floor. I must have crawled over to my recliner.

The paramedics got me to ER in time, but I was having a seizure in the ambulance, which the ER doctors noted and gave me a neuromuscular blocking drug. In fact, it was the same drug I had received for my Caesarian, and "I coded." So you guessed it—total respiratory failure and cardiac arrest. The heart paddles were needed again to resuscitate me.

This time I must have been immediately rejected by Heaven, because I didn't meet any of my relatives as I had when I met my father-in-law in 1986. I was in the hospital for five days, and I had a wallop of a headache. I also had a severe case of vertigo, but it came and went. Since the threat of falling again was very real, I was bed-ridden for all five days.

Dr. Freed prescribed special circulation leg sleeves that massaged my legs every so many minutes for several hours a day and night. He knew that bedridden PPS patients lose a lot of muscle strength very quickly. The longer I was in bed, the more loss would happen, and my strength as I knew it before the fall might never return. This time, I had suffered a major concussion and ended up with a traumatic brain injury (TBI).

After the hematoma in the lower right side of my brain started to go down, which many brain CT scans and MRI's showed, the neurologists noted at my release, in their medical opinion, I had an unremarkable brain that didn't require follow-up. I guess I should have taken that as a compliment at the time, but really...an *unremarkable* brain? Well they clearly didn't know me!

I was just so relieved to still have all my speech and reflexes intact. Many TBI patients cannot say the same. Once again, I said my gratitude prayer to God for such a blessing.

Due to my body going into total respiratory failure and cardiac arrest, I was diagnosed as a congestive heart failure patient. I was treated by cardiologists while in the hospital. Since I had never had a heart problem before, I refused to let them do invasive diagnostics on me. Dennis and I explained to the hospital cardiologists that I wanted to find my own heart doctor. I promised I would get into see one as soon as I was released.

It made all the difference in the world having Dennis by my side. He insisted on knowing whether or not the doctors felt I would be medically at risk if I delayed a heart catheterization, which was the invasive diagnostic procedure they wanted to do. When they answered that a short delay would be safe, Dennis spoke up and said, "Okay then, Dianne will find her own cardiologist, thank you." It didn't make the doctors happy, but they had to agree to my right to refuse. Nothing like having my own lawyer by my side.

There was another reason why I wanted to find my own heart doctor. I always engage in a partnership with all my doctors. I rely on establishing a mutual respect and good communication. I didn't feel that way toward this group of hospital cardiologists, and Dennis didn't either.

At one of their preliminary examinations of me, I told them, "The only reason I got hurt when I fell was because I was only drinking a smoothie. It should have been my favorite Irish whiskey. If it had been the whiskey, I wouldn't have gotten hurt." They didn't laugh. I knew I could never have them on my doctor list.

I did have to go to a hearing and balance doctor for the vertigo, which only got worse as time went on. He had a vertigo chair, which I call an astronaut chair. It treated severe cases of vertigo by strapping patients into the chair and then spinning them around in various horizontal and vertical positions. I was one of the lucky candidates for astronaut training and was strapped into the treatment chair. It worked after about twenty minutes. I was cured of vertigo, only to have it come back a week later. The vertigo doctor's office got me back into the chair ASAP, and my vertigo stopped with another twenty-minute session. That time vertigo ceased for good.

My TBI affected my eyesight and caused a traumatic cataract in my right eye, which was removed a year later. My hearing also declined, which my audiologist felt was due to having a TBI. Fortunately, I had already adjusted to having hearings aids in both ears several years before the concussion, so my hearing aids were adjusted to meet my needs now as a TBI patient.

The cardiac arrest that followed the concussion put my body in a long struggle back to breathing and moving normally. I had lost so much strength from being bedridden that I wondered if I would ever be able to live my life as I always had. I certainly was very dependent on Dennis. I hated being such a burden. I became quite depressed. I had many talks with God with questions like, "Now what?" My "can do" spirit had checked out. In all my previous challenges, I had overcome them, but this time was different. I had never felt more like giving up than I did then.

I was very blessed to know a wonderful woman named Brenda, from our church choir. She was a nurse for a very well-respected cardiology group in Orlando and had been working for them for over twenty years. Dennis and I agreed that Brenda would be a great resource in finding me a good heart specialist. The choir had been praying for me ever since they first heard of my fall, so when I called Brenda and explained I needed to be seen ASAP, she went right to work. She returned my call the same day I called her. Brenda made my appointment with one of their cardiologists. She told me that she had read my hospital file of my fall and had started to cry. She told me that it was a miracle I made it out of the hospital in only five days. Brenda knew me well from our choir time together, so she knew what a stubborn fighter I could be.

We had gotten to know each other quite well during the previous year's Fiftieth Jubilee Broadway Revue, when she was one of the lead stage hands. When it was my time to perform in the show, I came out on stage driving my scooter, while her husband followed behind me. He was dressed as the cowardly lion, and I was dressed as Dorothy from *The Wizard of Oz*.

Her husband had me giggling so hard before I had to sing *Somewhere Over the Rainbow*, I almost couldn't sing the song. Anyway, Brenda chose one of the best doctors in the practice for me, knowing that I would definitely click with his personality. She realized his medical knowledge was exactly what I needed to get my life back on track.

I had been put on blood pressure pills due to my blood pressure fluctuating drastically while in the hospital. I guess that's normal when a body is coding. I had never had blood pressure issues before, so my body was having a hard time adjusting. Thanks to my cardiologist telling me to keep a daily log, he was able to get me off the blood pressure pills safely. That helped my stamina to recuperate and heal much easier. It took over six months to reach a level of normalcy, but I kept telling myself I could heal. I also had to wait six months before I was allowed to drive again, since it was required by state law to be seizure-free for a full six months.

I knew the TBI had changed me. My sleep patterns had changed, and hearing was definitely affected. Not only were different levels of pitches and consonants hard to hear, but I found myself having a more difficult time filtering speech and ambient noise. My memory was more of a challenge when learning lyrics and new songs, and my sleep was interrupted with what later was diagnosed as restless leg syndrome. I was now dealing with my PPS fatigue, plus my new TBI body. Yes, I had always loved challenging circumstances, but this was not what I had bargained for. However, I used my music therapy to get back on the road to living, and within a year of that fateful fall, I was giving inspirational talks and performing for community groups again.

As time passed, I noticed PPS was definitely changing my life's boundaries. I had cut back on my musical activities and home duties. Dennis had taken over the vast majority of laundry and grocery shopping. My scoliosis was twisting my left shoulder and neck to a point that I couldn't even stretch it to the right without much effort and pain. Everyone ages at different rates, but at times I felt like I was in warp speed. The words of the orthopedic doctor that treated me in the 1980's and 90's came back to me in a whisper; "You may be this age, but your body is twenty years older." I figured I didn't have to like that fact, but I did have to live with these new issues and limitations now, which made me recognize and respect them. I set my goal to count my blessings, not my pains. I reminded myself that the doctors who treated me as an infant with polio, would never have believed I would be in my sixties, still performing and living life without any blood pressure pills or arthritis medication.

My cardiologist kept an annual eye on me and reassured me I didn't have heart disease. However, he agreed with me that my Vagus nerve was damaged by the polio virus. It affected my heart rhythm as well as many other parts of my anatomy. My heart rate raced occasionally and was a bit abnormal when compared with the majority of people. We agreed an annual checkup would be a good preventive strategy. Plus, he was such a nice man that I wanted to see him to catch up on life. I will always be grateful to Brenda for picking a perfect doctor for me.

In 2016, my friend Diane and I were asked to direct another Broadway Revue as a going- away surprise for the parish's associate priest Father George. Once again we two partners in "rhyme and crime" had a blast putting the show together. I had to memorize many songs for the show, so I started early on the task, since the TBI had changed my ability to memorize.

My singing abilities had changed too. I experienced much more weakness and fatigue. Since my scoliosis was curving more, my diaphragm muscle, which supports breath control, was being "squished" a bit. I knew my methods of musical phrasing had to change.

I chose *The Impossible Dream* as my solo number. I listened to several artists singing their interpretation of this popular Broadway song to see how they would sing certain phrases of it. Some artists sang the line, "To dream, the impossible dream," in only one solid breath, and others took a breath after "to dream," where the lyric had a comma. That's what I listened for in phrasing. I wondered if I could sing the musical phrases the way I wanted to, the way I felt them. I put all of my vocal technique and breath control training into big-time practice.

One of the joys that I have had being a music therapist, as well as a performer, is the singing and rehearsing of songs. Singing has always been what I love to do. The therapist in me has always known the therapeutic, physical exercise part of what I love to do. Singing increases my oxygen levels, which then feeds my entire body making memorizing and performing possible. I automatically prescribed my own music therapy prescription to keep living joyfully with my PPS changing body.

Dennis and I discussed how I could pace myself to conserve as much energy as possible with this new project. I decided to do the entire show in my scooter. In the past, I had only used my scooter for short parts. I always enjoyed blending into the group while standing with my cane for support. However, I was past blending in now. I embraced the blessing my scooter gave me, a gift of independence. Going into our partnership again, Diane knew that whenever I told her I couldn't make rehearsal she would totally support me saying, "The show must go on!" Let's face it, having a seasoned Broadway performer as a partner helped me conserve and preserve.

As always, I could not have been more supported by my family. Dennis took on cooking and cleanup many nights. Katie would call and check up on me, always saying her favorite mom lines, "Mom, are you being careful? Mom, are you sure you should be doing this?" They had picked me up off the floor too many times through the years. They could not help but be concerned with my Type-A personality performer being in charge of my decisions, instead of the wise, old polio survivor.

The show was a big success. When Dennis and I came home that evening, we both agreed I had balanced my activity level well, and he was proud of me. I was very tired that night. Also, I had started getting a cold the day before the show, but I sang through it. I knew I would sleep well, in spite of it. I woke up early the next morning, which is not my normal night owl routine, and got up with Dennis who has always been a morning person. I was just coming out to sit down in my recliner as Seamus came running in from being let outside for his morning potty break. In his excitement seeing me, he ran and jumped up on me, and down I went. (I KNOW what you are thinking…the dog again? What can I say? Love is blind and I'M NUTS.) I knew when I landed on my left knee, I had broken my kneecap again.

With Dennis's help, I managed to get up and then prayed to stay calm. I told Dennis where my old cast was, so he went and got it. We knew the healing routine of falls: ice pack, elevate leg, and homeopathic remedies for swelling and pain. It was a Saturday morning, so I refused to go to an emergency room, and I convinced Dennis I'd wait to see if Dr. Freed could see me on Monday. Dennis didn't like waiting because he saw how much pain I was in, but as usual he respected my choice.

Dr. Freed saw me that Monday afternoon and sent me for X-rays to confirm the break. He then told me I had to go to an orthopedic knee specialist for treatment. He knew how much I hated going to an orthopedic specialist, because most of them loved to prescribe surgery. I call them orthopedic specialists here, because after all they are specialists in orthopedics—in bones and muscles, joints and ligaments and how they all go together. However, they are also called orthopedic *surgeons*, or even "orthopods," for short.

I knew I was not a candidate for surgery, even if it was a possibility. However, Dr. Freed knew that too. I trusted his recommendation and advice, but I shared my feelings that I didn't want another doctor. I asked Dr. Freed if this new orthopod would just be a talker and not listen to me, or if I would be treated as a person who really knew my own body. I didn't want to be just another orthopedic case with symptoms. He assured me that she would listen to me and I would like her. I went to see her the next day.

Dr. Freed was right; I did like her. She knew that I had been through the fractured kneecap routine twice before, so she refreshed my memory with the do's and don'ts. She told me that in any other case, she would have me in surgery with a pin in my kneecap, but she could see that I wasn't just any other case. Once again, I was blessed with a conservative orthopedic physician. I thought to myself that Dr. Ponseti, who died in 2009, was looking out for me from heaven above, and I smiled to myself.

The treatment lasted eight weeks. I went back to the orthopedic doctor two more times during the eight-week recovery time. She was easy to talk to, and her conservative approach worked like a charm. My kneecap healed. She marveled at how the X-ray could hardly make out the image of my kneecap, due to it having very little bone mass. However, she told me to be extra careful, because my osteoporosis in that kneecap was very severe and it would break if I ever fell on it again. I assured her that I was changing my first name to Careful.

During my treatment, she had learned that I was once a Dr. Ponseti patient. I remembered her eyes widened when I mentioned his name, and she said, "What? You don't mean THE Ignacio Ponseti?" I nodded yes, and she went on to say, "Do you know what he did to the practice of orthopedics? He changed the entire philosophy, by showing that surgery was not always the correct treatment. Wow, no wonder you have done so well. You were treated by the best!" I told her what Dr. Ponseti always knew—that I Could! At my final appointment with her, I handed her a copy of a letter that Dr. Ponseti wrote to me describing my history with him. She said, "Oh my goodness, can I keep this?" I said, "I made you that copy to keep." I was so thrilled that she knew of and respected Dr. Ponseti, so the letter was something I wanted her to have.

It turned out that it was very lucky I liked the orthopedic doctor. Ten months later, in May 2018, I fell again on my left knee. No, it wasn't the dog that caused the fall this time!

I had just gone for my swim. Exercise in the pool was my safest way to exercise, but even being safe, it brought a level of PPS fatigue. So all it took was stubbing my toe on a section of the doorway as I walked to my lift-chair—and down I went. Katie had come over for a Sunday dinner visit that day, so she and Dennis were right there in the room as I fell. They rushed to pick me up off the floor. Katie helped me balance on my right leg, while Dennis went to get the wheelchair we kept for emergencies. I waited until the next morning to call Dr. Freed.

After telling Dr. Freed that I had fallen on the kneecap again, he told me to get into the same knee specialist as before, ASAP. I was able to see her that same week. She just shook her head, smiling at me as she entered the examining room and said, "Well, I knew that I liked having you as a patient of mine, but I certainly didn't think I'd see you back so soon." That sentiment was very mutual, but there I was. I agreed to behave and follow the same treatment guidelines as before. She said that she would see me in four weeks.

My PPS was definitely increasing. I tired much faster than ever before, doing very little physical activity. Walking was harder, and it started to become scarier to me. I knew I couldn't let fear rule my life, but the fear of falling was very real. My faith was grounded in believing I was always protected by God, but I had to dig deeper into my soul to get through these new life limitations.

Back in the year 2001, I had learned to practice a daily, alternative form of self-healing treatment called energy medicine. One of my dear friends, Maggie, had learned of a conference teaching energy medicine. She was a certified massage therapist and had watched my body get weaker in the fifteen years she had known me. She suggested I attend the conference with her, so that together we could learn an alternative way to help my body maintain its strength. Once again, God put the right person, Maggie, in my life so that I would keep living my "I Could" attitude.

That conference began a lifetime practice that supported my belief in the power of self-healing. It is a combination of ancient Chinese medicine principles, which explain the meridian systems of the body, along with ancient Indian health principles, which explain the chakra system of the body. Energy medicine also included a psychological approach to meditation. In my case, I adapted the principles of energy medicine techniques into a form of daily prayer.

Since my PPS weakness was increasing along with many more falls, I decided to look for a certified energy healer while recuperating from my kneecap fracture. I had been receiving monthly newsletters for years from the teacher who had led the conference Maggie and I had attended years earlier. She had resources on her webpage to locate certified healers in many areas of the United States. I found one listed only nine miles away from my house. The energy healer had been trained and certified by the conference teacher herself.

I went for my first session a week after I first saw my orthopedic doctor, where the X-rays revealed the degree of fracture in my kneecap. The degree would require a full eight to ten weeks for complete healing. I described the fracture to the energy healer, as well as the history of my three previous ones. I had the leg brace on which was a leg immobilizer, and I transferred from my scooter onto her massage table. After her history intake of me, where I described my PPS as well as the pain I felt in my arthritic joints, she described a treatment plan for my body to increase its energy flow. She also mentioned some homeopathic remedies I might be interested in trying. The session lasted an hour and a half. Dennis was waiting in the parking lot to drive me home. He could tell I felt better, and I assured him I did.

Each day I practiced the energy medicine techniques prescribed for me. There were days when I practiced the movements more than once a day. I purchased one of the homeopathic remedies and began taking it twice a day. I saw the energy healer again ten days after my initial session. Once again, I felt less pain after the session, especially in my neck. Now you might think that the sessions included massage, but they did not. In fact, the energy healer barely touched any part of my body. Since I had been a student of energy medicine techniques for over fifteen years, I was able to work with her in a way that helped direct her methodology. As with every health provider I have ever had, we were a team that worked together on my healing.

Soon after, I went to a scheduled four-week checkup with my knee specialist, the orthopedic doctor. New X-rays were taken to see if my fracture was starting to heal back together. Since I had been through this three times before, I knew the progress was slow. I hoped that whatever was revealed on the X-ray images it would clearly be progress.

My doctor was surprised to see that my fracture was healing faster than the one she had treated the previous year. She told me that whatever I was doing, I was doing it well and to keep it up. I didn't tell her about my energy medicine and homeopathic remedies. I have found from experience that the majority of MD's don't believe in using homeopathic remedies, let alone energy medicine. However, I was blessed with Dr. Freed because he had gotten certified in acupuncture, where he had studied the principles of Chinese medicine meridian systems. I left the appointment with my doctor very pleased, and I agreed to keep healing. I would see her in another four weeks.

My kneecap healed completely in eight weeks, and I was released from my doctor's care. She and I made a pact that we would not see each other again...well, at least not in less than a year! I continued with several more energy healing sessions with my energy healer. Each session taught me more techniques to keep healing my body. Finally, she and I agreed that I had enough knowledge to continue my energy healing routine on my own at home. I knew that if I ever felt the need for a "tune-up," she was only a phone call away.

I went to see Dr. Freed after my knee had healed in July 2017. "Even with all my self-healing and serious conservation methods to keep my strength, I feel like I've hit a major plateau," I told him. "Now I'm spiraling downward. Think it's time to get a powerchair, so I can walk less and conserve energy." My scooter, due to its size, was never functional enough inside the house. A power wheelchair would be.

He looked me squarely in the eye and asked, "Are you sure you're ready for this?"

I didn't hesitate. "More than ready."

We discussed that, if I gave up walking permanently, I would lose the ability to walk. "I'll work out how to balance my walking and my rolling without increasing the threat of falling. As a musician," I told him, "I'll figure out how to 'walk & roll' to my own beat."

Dr. Freed smiled and advised me that the next step would be a physical therapy evaluation. As the director of the hospital's rehabilitation department he oversaw all the physical therapists. He sent my therapy prescription to one of the centers that dealt with neurological rehab issues.

The supervisor of physical therapists, Linda, along with a medical equipment vendor named Art, evaluated me for my new powerchair. They measured me and took me through the paces, noting various range-of-motion issues, as well as strengths and deficits.

The result: yes, I would qualify for a specialized Powerchair. I assumed it would be like many of the chairs my PPS friends used.

I was shocked when Art went out to his van and brought in a POWERCHAIR! It looked like a robot that came out of a sci-fi movie. I had only seen chairs like this for our wounded veterans who had lost limbs, or for para- or quadriplegics, but I didn't see myself like that. Am I that bad?

Linda said "Go ahead and sit in it, Dianne. See how it feels."

The minute I lowered myself into the powerchair, I said, "Oh my God, this is the most comfortable chair I have ever sat in. I feel like my whole body is supported."

Linda said, "Try tilting the seat back," and Art showed me how.

Right away, the reclining angle took the pressure off my spine and torso and neck. "I'm glad the headrest supports my neck as well. I don't feel the strain of holding my head up that I've always felt—in any seated position."

Art said, "Let me show you how to raise the legs of the chair so you can recline."

"Good idea," Linda said. "Reclining will help your circulation." After I'd worked the controls into that position and back again, she said, "I have something else to show you that I think you're going to like."

More than liking it, I loved this final thing she showed me the most: the chair could be raised up a full ten to twelve inches. Suddenly, I was at eye level with people standing. I felt God smiling at me, guiding me through this whole new experience. Suddenly I forgot about my fears and doubts about my declining strength. I said, "Now, this chair will take care of my body, the temple that God made." I can't wait to learn how to live fully with my new wheels.

I was like a kid at Christmas, driving the powerchair up and down the therapy center halls. I couldn't help but drive it as fast as it could go because it was much faster than my scooter ever was. Art and Linda just watched and laughed at me as my speed-demon reputation took over.

"I can't wait for my own chair. How soon can it be ordered?" I asked.

They glanced at one another and told me to be patient. Linda said, "Sometimes it takes from six months to a year for the processing and insurance approvals to be completed. But we'll get started. I'll send my evaluation to Dr. Freed."

"Once he approves it," Art said, "I'll handle the prescription and ordering."

I left the evaluation feeling so very blessed. My limitations weren't forcing me into a wheelchair but introducing me to wonderful new possibilities of independence and better health.

By August 2018, I was asked to take over the children's choir at my parish. Dennis and I discussed how I could accomplish it without doing more harm to my changing body. As always, Dennis was all in favor of it. He told me he would fix supper on the Thursday evenings when I had weekly rehearsals.

My powerchair had been approved by my insurance and it would really help me directing the children's rehearsals and performances. I continued to feel more pain—much more than ever before—in my neck and in my left ribcage area. Almost everything I did became more of a challenge. I had always adapted my body to accomplish things most people never think about, and now my learned adaptations were hurting me. I was very careful directing each week with my children's choir, but I still felt new pains.

Meanwhile, driving my van was getting harder. My range of motion for turning my head was much more restrictive. I wondered how I could see traffic. I continued to fight my fears, and with the Christmas Mass schedule coming up, I had to prepare carefully to conserve to preserve. But I knew it was probably time to have a checkup.

I made the appointment with Dr. Freed in November. It was the first appointment I had since my powerchair had been delivered, and he beamed at me. "I'm so happy you have the chair now. Let me see you maneuver it." I demonstrated how I got in and out of the chair, and I drove in and out of the various examining rooms, as well as into his office, where he said, "I'm quite impressed. You didn't take off any part of the doorways on the way in and out of the rooms."

During my checkup evaluation, I described the new pain and stiffness in my neck. He said, "I'm prescribing that you return to physical therapy with Linda again. If the pain gets worse, I would recommend giving you a cortisone shot in the neck." I agreed but said, "I'd like to try Linda first."

The following week, Linda evaluated my new neck pain and designed an exercise program to stretch my neck safely and increase my range of motion. I went three times a week faithfully, hoping to feel better by Christmastime. The stretching exercises hurt, but they also helped.

I made it through the Christmas rush and demands at the church, and I was very proud of the children in the choir. However, on the Saturday three days after Christmas, I bent over in order to reach and scratch my nose and doubled up with a pain I had never felt before. Somehow, my right shoulder had come out of the socket.

What should I do? I can't go to the ER. Experience had taught me that most emergency doctors are shocked to see how my body is put together. Going to an ER would only make it worse. Besides, I had a physical therapy appointment the following Monday. I decided I would let them evaluate it and report back to Dr. Freed.

In the meantime, I tried to position myself in my lift chair to see if I could get the shoulder back into place. After several hours of trying everything I could, it somehow slipped back into position. I was so relieved—of both pain and of fear.

I never thought my shoulders would ever be any problem, since I could never raise them or use my arms like others. However, my adapting to life put wear and tear on the joints that didn't have deltoid and other arm muscles to support them. I never thought about how I threw my arms—one holding the other—in order to reach, grab, lift, and even wash myself.

It isn't until we lose something that we realize how our life has changed. I used to say that, since I was born with polio, I didn't know what I had lost since I never had it to begin with. Life had now changed that for me. Now, I felt the loss. I also felt sorry for myself. However, I knew that if I kept up with my pity party I couldn't expect to heal and live my life as fully as I wanted.

I dug deep into my soul and practiced my prayerful meditation techniques. I made a vow to myself and God above to overcome my self-pity and fear. I had to begin a huge practice of surrendering to God's plan for me. I also knew that fear never comes from God. I tapped into my wonderful Divine Healer while listening to the voices of all my supportive family, teachers, friends, and yes, even my doctors, who I knew had become my friends. All of them were saying I could.

EPILOGUE

It has taken me nearly five years to write my story. Many health issues during these years have resulted in further loss of abilities, ones that I never thought I'd face. I have had more falls since my legs are getting much weaker. Walking is more of a challenge and more of a risk, because my arms cannot support me with a cane or a walker. I have shed some tears. However, these past five years have brought many successes, joys and laughter too. I still thank God for my power-chair each day.

I was born during the polio epidemic, and I sure don't plan on going out of this world during a pandemic! My self-care healing techniques and faith are being put to great use.

I am now experiencing the same relief the world felt when the polio vaccine was discovered and distributed. I can now relate to my parents' feelings of relief when they were finally vaccinated for polio. I have no doubt they sent many prayers of thanksgiving to our Heavenly God.

When I wrote these words, COVID-19 vaccination appointments were very hard to secure, but I believed that I would get my coronavirus vaccine at the right time. Once again, God was giving me opportunities galore to practice patience. I will keep doing my part in securing my future vaccination appointments, since I have many goals to complete and plans for living life as fully as possible.

I am still dealing with my shoulder joints and pain. Both are very arthritic, but my right shoulder is the only one that occasionally pops out of place. With my adaptive talents, combined with super care from Dennis and excellent medical care from Dr. Freed, I am able to live a blessed life.

Sometimes sacrifices are forced upon me by my body controlling what I can and cannot do. These sacrifices occur much more than they ever did before. I occasionally struggle with some of those limits, such as never playing the guitar again. I do miss it. However, the pain of popping my shoulder out of its socket happens to be a very high motivator in the acceptance of giving up the guitar.

On the other hand, I constantly remind myself that I am still blessed with being able to go to the bathroom by myself.

I don't take normal routines for granted, with some being more challenging than others. I keep facing each day with faith and hope. Someone recently asked me why I didn't call my challenges "struggles." I replied that if I started my days thinking about struggles, I probably wouldn't want to get out of bed. I will never like dealing with PPS, but I do respect it, and I try to face it realistically every day.

I am using my powerchair every day, along with balancing my life with careful walking and leg exercise. "Arthur," my arthritis-laden mother's nickname for arthritis, is in most of my joints. As Mom used to say, "If I wasn't going steady with Arthur, I'd feel great!"

I am very pleased that I am not on any medication for high blood pressure or heart disease or cholesterol, which many sixty-eight-year-olds have been on for years. Although I have had to get a cortisone shot in my shoulder, mostly I am on supplements and vitamins. I continue to believe in and practice daily energy healing and meditative prayer, conduits to a powerful source of energy.

And I still sing and use my gifts of music and occasionally compose hymns and songs.

During this time of COVID-19, I am isolating as much as possible in order to stay healthy, but I find myself searching for new distance-learning experiences. I love learning. I utilize online classes in many different areas, from music recording to philosophy to natural healing and much more. Still, I am quite content sitting in my powerchair, conserving my energy and strength.

Balancing the joy and sadness of life is a constant for all of us. I love the days that are filled with laughter, yet some are filled with tears. I accept each day as it comes, knowing it's a gift of possibilities. Each gives me another opportunity to master the art of life. I am always being carried by my Friend and Master from above.

We all have our own belief systems that help us live. One of my beliefs is that we manifest what we think. I believe nature provides a perfect setting for the manifestation of the majesty this world can be. Maintaining a beautiful vision of the world keeps me grounded in positive energy, which I believe comes straight from God above. With Him, I can face anything.

As I face new physical, spiritual, and mental trials, I find my backyard is a haven of strength. We have many hawks and backyard birds, squirrels, snakes, opossums and an occasional armadillo. Now, I grant you that snakes aren't my favorite creatures, but I have acquired an admiration for their stealth-like grace—as long as they do it outside and not in my garage, under my van, or on my porch.

Nature is an abundant healing source open to all of us. Even if you don't have a nature setting readily available, there are superb nature videos online. You can immerse yourself in a world of beautiful settings. The videos with peaceful background music playing are my favorites. The double sensory gifts, seeing nature and listening to music at the same time, can't be beat.

Even though I know aging with PPS is accelerating my physical health issues, I believe what I was taught years ago: I will be able to do things my way. I live as Dr. Freed suggested on one of my recent appointments, "Dianne, from now on everything you do has to be measured with a level of risk involved." That is not an easy thing to do for a person like me, but I know I am learning how each day. Somedays I am better at it than on other days, but I know I must live with measured risk in order to live *my way.* If I find I can't do it my way, independently, I will find help. And it will come from all the loving people in my life. There is nothing like family and friends. I know I am not alone in this world. I have been blessed with faith in God the Father, the Son, and the Holy Spirit. That faith confirms my life's lessons each and every moment I live.

We are all here to help each other live good lives. The simple truth is that we all have the same two choices when we wake up each day: Are you going to be happy and make others happy today, or are you going to be miserable and make everyone else miserable, too?

That is the simple truth I tell myself each and every day. On some days though, factors like pain can twist that simple truth into a big challenge. However, I make my day's first choice of being happy much easier to make, by simply finding things to be grateful for. Some days the pain does not go away, but it is much more bearable with an "attitude of gratitude."

And I believe I have been given the biggest gift of all: the gift of God's love. He made sure my life's lessons would be surrounded by His love. My Lord put the "somebodies" in my life—somebodies who believed enough in me that I was able to learn to believe in me, too. What gets me through my life are the memories of those somebodies from my past, along with the somebodies I still have in my life today: my family and friends.

When people ask me, "How do you do it, Dianne?" I can honestly say, "Because somebody told me I could!"

-The End-

ABOUT THE AUTHOR

Dianne Wall is a recording artist, music therapist, music educator, and motivational speaker from Winter Springs, Florida. She received her BA in Music Education and a Masters of Music Therapy degree from Florida State University, Tallahassee. She has been a featured soloist in Europe and all over the United States. She was a music therapist for 10 years in area schools. Dianne has been a church director of music, as well as the music director for the premiere production of Historic Sanford's community theater. She has professionally recorded in area recording studios, and sings in a variety of venues. She released an inspirational CD *Touched by the Light* in 2000, which includes "Mary's Song," one of her own compositions. She incorporates her voice and her love of music therapy in her motivational speaking engagements. Dianne tells her life experience of being born with polio, and now living with post polio syndrome. Her personal story explains how her faith provides the strength and direction which she has depended on throughout her entire life. She loves to share her "can do" attitude with others, hoping it inspires many to go out and make a difference.

Made in the USA
Monee, IL
25 January 2024